Ernst Schering Research Foundation Workshop 19
EGF Receptor in Tumor Growth and Progression

Springer-Verlag Berlin Heidelberg GmbH

Ernst Schering Research Foundation
Workshop 19

EGF Receptor in Tumor Growth and Progression

R.B. Lichtner, R.N. Harkins
Editors

With 63 Figures in 100 Separate Illustrations
and 18 Tables

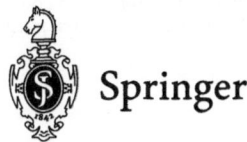 Springer

Series Editors: G. Stock and U.-F. Habenicht

CIP data applied for

Die Deutsche Bibliothek – CIP-Einheitsaufnahme
Schering-Forschungsgesellschaft <Berlin>: Ernst Schering Research Foundation
Workshop. – Berlin; Heidelberg; New York; Barcelona; Budapest; Hong Kong; London;
Milan; Paris; Santa Clara; Singapore; Tokyo: Springer.
ISSN 0947-6075
NE: HST
19. EGF receptor in tumor growth and progression. – 1997
EGF receptor in tumor growth and progression / R.B. Lichtner and R.N. Harkins ed. –
Berlin; Heidelberg; New York; Barcelona; Budapest; Hong Kong; London; Milan; Paris;
Santa Clara; Singapore; Tokyo: Springer, 1997
(Ernst Schering Research Foundation Workshop; 19)

ISBN 978-3-662-03393-7   ISBN 978-3-662-03391-3 (eBook)
DOI 10.1007/978-3-662-03391-3

NE: Litchner R.B. [Hrsg.]

Originally published by Springer-Verlag Berlin Heidelberg New York in 1997

Softcover reprint of the hardcover 1st edition 1997

21/3135–5 4 3 2 1 0 – Printed on acid-free paper

Preface

The last 15 years have brought an understanding of growth and differentiation at the molecular level, expanding our knowledge of the origin and progression of cancer. Early breakthroughs defining growth control pathways came via studies of oncogenes, mutated signaling molecules that have lost the capacity to turn off their proliferative signal. Oncogenes with diverse growth-promoting activities have been discovered, covering the gamut from cell surface to nuclear signaling. Sequencing of these oncogenes revealed that they were mutated forms of captured cellular genes and displayed tyrosine kinase activity. The epidermal growth factor (EGF) receptor was the first of 40–50 transmembrane tyrosine kinase receptors to be cloned and sequenced. Beyond cell proliferation, activation of EGF receptor by its specific ligands controls important physiological processes, such as cell differentiation, apoptosis, cell migration, and cell shape. Activation of autocrine growth loops, consisting in solid human tumors of upregulated expression of EGFR together with increased production of ligands suggested its crucial role in autonomous tumor growth.

This workshop provided an opportunity to bring together basic and clinical research scientists to discuss new avenues for therapies directed at the EGF receptor and its associated signaling and regulatory systems. A broad range of topics on EGF receptor biology were presented, including the regulation of signaling by phosphatases, role of heterodimerization, tumor growth and metastasis in animal models, clinical studies, and the status of current strategies to target the EGF receptor with monoclonal antibodies for tumor therapy. We hope that this book with its detailed analysis of EGF receptor signal transduction

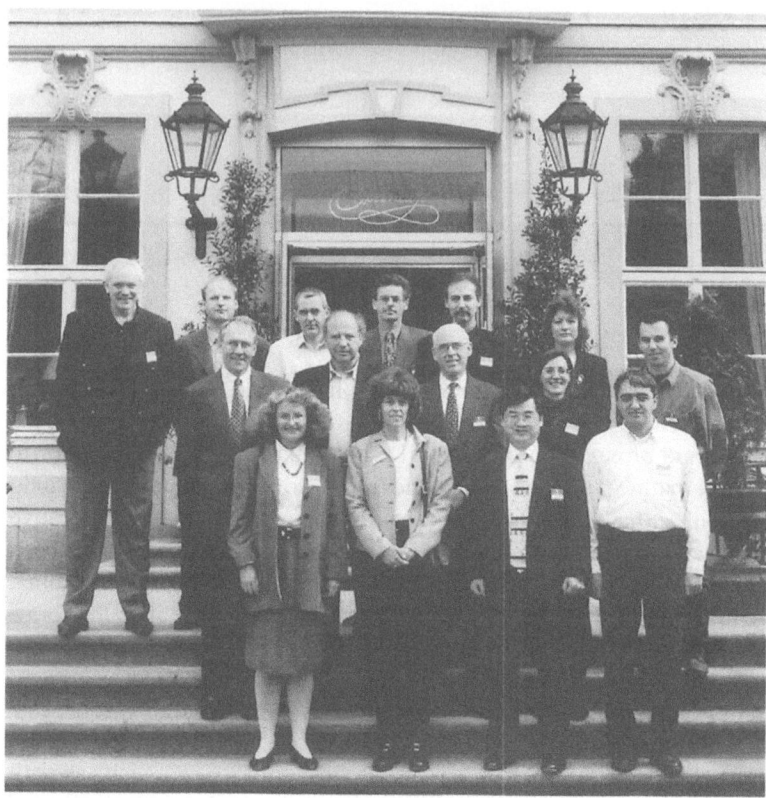

The participants of the workshop. *From left to right; first row:* R.B. Lichtner,
N.E. Hynes, D.M. Shin, K. Khazaie; *second row:* R.N. Harkins, M. Klagsbrun,
J. Mendelsohn, S.A. Chrysogelos, F. Radvanyi; *third row:* R.I. Nicholson,
W. Wels, F.-D. Böhmer, M.R. Schneider, A.L. Harris, S.A. Eccles

via expression of receptor, ligands, phosphatases and presence of other
members of the receptor family will provide valuable information for
the development of novel therapeutic interventions.

R.B. Lichtner
R.N. Harkins

Table of Contents

List of Editors and Contributors

Editors

R.B. Lichtner
Research Laboratories of Schering AG, Experimental Oncology,
Müllerstraße 178, 13342 Berlin, Germany

R.N. Harkins
Berlex Biosciences, Protein Biochemistry and Biophysics,
Richmond, CA 94804-0099, USA

Contributors

G. Allison
Departments of Surgery and Pathology, Children's Hospital,
Harvard Medical School, Boston, MA 02115, USA

M. Barth
Lombardi Cancer Center and the Department of Biochemistry and Molecular
Biology, E407 TRB, Georgetown University, 3970 Reservoir Rd., NW,
Washington, DC 20007, USA

J. Baselga
Memorial Sloan-Kettering Cancer Center, New York, NY 10021, USA

R.R. Beerli
Friedrich Miescher Institute, P.O. Box 2543, 4002 Basel, Switzerland

S. Bellusci
UMR 144 CNRS - Institut Curie, Institut Curie Research Division,
26 rue d'Ulm, 75248 Paris Cedex 05, France

F.-D. Böhmer
Max-Planck Society, Research Unit "Molecular Cell Biology",
Medical Faculty, Friedrich-Schiller University, Drackendorfer Str. 1,
07747 Jena, Germany

G. Box
Section of Immunology, McElwain Laboratories, Institute of Cancer
Research, Cotswold Road, Belmont, Sutton, Surrey SM2 5NG, UK

B. Boyer
UMR 144 CNRS - Institut Curie, Institut Curie Research Division,
26 rue d'Ulm, 75248 Paris Cedex 05, France

C. Brown
Memorial Sloan-Kettering Cancer Center, New York, NY 10021, USA

S.A. Chrysogelos
Lombardi Cancer Center and the Department of Biochemistry and Molecular
Biology, E407 TRB, Georgetown University, 3970 Reservoir Rd., NW,
Washington, DC 20007, USA

J.L. Chou
Memorial Sloan-Kettering Cancer Center, New York, NY 10021, USA

W. Court
Section of Immunology, McElwain Laboratories, Institute of Cancer
Research, Cotswold Road, Belmont, Sutton, Surrey SM2 5NG, UK

S.K. Das
Physiology and Obstetrics and Gynecology,
University of Kansas Medical Center, Kansas City, KS 66160, USA

C. Dean
Section of Immunology, McElwain Laboratories, Institute of Cancer
Research, Cotswold Road, Belmont, Sutton, Surrey SM2 5NG, UK

S.K. Dey
Departments of Physiology and Obstetrics and Gynecology,
University of Kansas Medical Center, Kansas City, KS 66160, USA

S.A. Eccles
Section of Immunology, McElwain Laboratories, Institute of Cancer
Research, Cotswold Road, Belmont, Sutton, Surrey SM2 5NG, UK

K. Elenius
Departments of Surgery and Pathology, Children's Hospital,
Harvard Medical School, Boston, MA 02115, USA

Z. Fan
Memorial Sloan-Kettering Cancer Center, New York, NY 10021, USA

J.M.W. Gee
Tenovus Cancer Research Centre, University of Wales College of Medicine,
Cardiff, UK

B. Groner
Institute for Experimental Cancer Research, Tumor Biology Center,
Breisacher Str. 117, 79106 Freiburg, Germany

R.N. Harkins
Berlex Biosciences, Protein Biochemistry and Biophysics,
Richmond, CA 94804-0099, USA

M.E. Harper
Tenovus Cancer Research Centre, University of Wales College of Medicine,
Cardiff, UK

A.L. Harris
ICRF Molecular Oncology Laboratories, University of Oxford,
Institute of Molecular Medicine, John Radcliffe Hospital, Oxford OX3 9DU

W.N. Hittelman
Department of Clinical Investigation, The University of Texas
M. D. Anderson Cancer Center, 1515 Holcombe Boulevard, Box 80,
Houston, TX 77030, USA

M. Hoffmann
Institute for Experimental Cancer Research, Tumor Biology Center,
Breisacher Str. 117, 79106 Freiburg, Germany

W.K. Hong
Department of Thoracic/Head and Neck Medical Oncology,
The University of Texas M. D. Anderson Cancer Center,
1515 Holcombe Boulevard, Box 80, Houston, TX 77030, USA

N.E. Hynes
Friedrich Miescher Institute, P.O. Box 2543, 4002 Basel, Switzerland

M. Jeschke
Friedrich Miescher Institute, P.O. Box 2543, 4002 Basel, Switzerland

J. Jouanneau
UMR 144 CNRS - Institut Curie, Institut Curie Research Division,
26 rue d'Ulm, 75248 Paris Cedex 05, France

K. Khazaie
Institut für Immunologie, Deutsches Krebsforschungszentrum,
Im Neuenheimer Feld 280, 69120 Heidelberg, Germany

M. Klagsbrun
Departments of Surgery and Pathology, Children's Hospital,
Harvard Medical School, Boston, MA 02115, USA

R.B. Lichtner
Research Laboratories of Schering AG, Experimental Oncology,
Müllerstraße 178, 13342 Berlin, Germany

H. Masui
Memorial Sloan-Kettering Cancer Center, New York, NY 10021, USA

J. Mendelsohn
M.D. Anderson Cancer Center, 1515 Holcombe Boulevard,
Houston, TX 77030, USA

H. Modjtahedi
Section of Immunology, McElwain Laboratories, Institute of Cancer
Research, Cotswold Road, Belmont, Sutton, Surrey SM2 5NG, UK

R.I. Nicholson
Tenovus Cancer Research Centre, University of Wales College of Medicine,
Cardiff CF4 4XX, UK

B.C. Paria
Physiology and Obstetrics and Gynecology,
University of Kansas Medical Center, Kansas City, KS 66160, USA

D. Peng
Memorial Sloan-Kettering Cancer Center, New York, NY 10021, USA

R. Perez-Soler
Department of Thoracic/Head and Neck Medical Oncology,
The University of Texas M. D. Anderson Cancer Center,
1515 Holcombe Boulevard, Box 80, Houston, TX 77030, USA

F. Radvanyi
UMR 144 CNRS - Institut Curie, Institut Curie Research Division,
26 rue d'Ulm, 75248 Paris Cedex 05, France

J.F.R. Robertson
Department of Surgery, City Hospital, Nottingham, UK

P. Savagner
UMR 144 CNRS - Institut Curie, Institut Curie Research Division,
26 rue d'Ulm, 75248 Paris Cedex 05, France

M. Schmidt
Institute for Experimental Cancer Research, Tumor Biology Center,
Breisacher Str. 117, 79106 Freiburg, Germany

D.M. Shin
Department of Thoracic/Head and Neck Medical Oncology,
The University of Texas M. D. Anderson Cancer Center,
1515 Holcombe Boulevard, Box 80, Houston, TX 77030, USA

J.P. Thiery
UMR 144 CNRS - Institut Curie, Institut Curie Research Division,
26 rue d'Ulm, 75248 Paris Cedex 05, France

J. Titley
Section of Immunology, McElwain Laboratories, Institute of Cancer
Research, Cotswold Road, Belmont, Sutton, Surrey SM2 5NG, UK

A.M. Vallés
UMR 144 CNRS - Institut Curie, Institut Curie Research Division,
26 rue d'Ulm, 75248 Paris Cedex 05, France

A.E. Wakeling
Zeneca Pharmaceuticals, Macclesfield, UK

W. Wels
Institute for Experimental Cancer Research, Tumor Biology Center,
Breisacher Str. 117, 79106 Freiburg, Germany

P. Willsher
Department of Surgery, City Hospital, Nottingham, UK

M.A. Wilson
Lombardi Cancer Center and the Department of Biochemistry and Molecular
Biology, E407 TRB, Georgetown University, 3970 Reservoir Rd., NW,
Washington, DC 20007, USA

X. Wu
Memorial Sloan-Kettering Cancer Center, New York, NY 10021, USA

R.I. Yarden
Lombardi Cancer Center and the Department of Biochemistry and Molecular
Biology, E407 TRB, Georgetown University, 3970 Reservoir Rd., NW,
Washington, DC 20007, USA

1 Signal Transduction by EGF Receptor Tyrosine Kinase

R.B. Lichtner and R.N. Harkins

1.1 Introduction

Members of the receptor tyrosine kinase family are frequently implicated in experimental models of neoplasia as well as in human cancer.
One of the best studied receptor signaling systems from this family is
the epidermal growth factor receptor (EGFR). The EGFR is widely
expressed in mammals and has been implicated in various stages of
embryonic development. Recently, EGFR knockout mice by targeted
disruption of exon 1 (Sibilia and Wagner 1995) or exon 2 (Miettinen et
al. 1995; Threadgill et al. 1995) of the mouse EGFR gene have been
reported. The resulting phenotypes of EGFR$^{-/-}$ embryos or newborns

were very similar. Growth retardation and epithelial immaturity were found, with the severity of defects being dependent on the mouse genetic background. These results indicate that the EGFR is of fundamental importance in the regulation of epithelial proliferation and differentiation. Experiments with transgenic mice suggest that an autocrine mechanism involving the EGFR could be expected to play a role in the initiation and/or progression of tumors. Transgenic mice expressing transforming growth factor-α (TGF-α) were reported to develop mammary and hepatocellular carcinoma as well as pancreatic hyperplasia (Jhappan et al. 1990; Sandgreen et al. 1990). Evidently, none of these neoplasias required amplification or truncation of the EGFR, but rather depended on the paracrine activation of the endogenous receptor. In human tumors, abnormal receptor signaling has been assigned to over-expression of receptor or ligand or truncated forms of receptor, which are observed in some forms of neoplastic development. The EGFR is overexpressed in many tumors of epithelial origin, including glioblas-toma and cancers of the lung, breast, head and neck, and bladder (Gul-lick 1991). A closely related receptor, erbB-2, is also amplified or overexpressed in a large number of adenocarcinomas, including breast, ovary, lung, stomach, and salivary gland (Hynes 1993). Furthermore, studies have shown that patients with tumors showing overexpression of the EGFR or erbB-2 have a poor prognosis (Sainsbury et al. 1987; Slamon et al. 1987; Nicholson et al. 1988). Thus the elevated levels of these receptors coupled with their location at the surface of the cell render them good drug targets for cancer therapies.

1.2 Receptor Structure

The EGFR is a 170-kDa glycoprotein translated from mRNAs of 6 and 10 kb encoded by a gene on chromosome 7q21. The mature human EGFR is a single polypeptide chain of 1186 amino acids, which traverses the plasma membrane with a single hydrophobic anchor sequence. The receptor is composed of a large extracellular ligand-binding domain, a single transmembrane region, and a cytoplasmic portion with a conserved protein tyrosine kinase domain and a carboxy-terminal tail that contains the autophosphorylation sites (Ullrich and Schlessinger 1990). The extracellular amino terminal end can be divided into four domains, with the third domain being responsible for high-affinity binding to EGF and other specific ligands of the receptor. At least two cytoplasmic regions, the juxtamembrane and carboxy-terminal domains, are targets for phosphorylation by protein kinase C (PKC; on serine residues) or cross phosphorylation by EGFR (on tyrosine residues). Changes in phosphorylation regulate the affinity for ligand as well as the activity and specificity of the protein tyrosine kinase function. Binding of ATP to the lysine at position 721 within the EGFR kinase domain is the key event required to initiate tyrosine kinase activity of the receptor.

The cell surface EGFR population constitutes of at least two receptor subclasses with different ligand-binding affinity, a minor high- and major low-affinity subclass. The differences in ligand-binding affinity are probably not due to the primary structure of both receptor subclasses, since transfection of cells exhibiting no EGFR with an expression vector containing a single EGFR gene results in expression of both high- and low-affinity receptors.

1.3 Receptor Activation

1.3.1 Ligands

The first known specific ligand for the EGFR was EGF/urogastrone, which has a proliferative effect on epidermal cells expressing the receptor. The family of EGF-like growth factors known to bind to the EGFR includes TGF-α, amphiregulin, heparin-binding EGF, betacellulin, epiregulin, and a number of virally encoded peptides (schwannoma-derived growth factor, vaccinia growth factor, shapes fibroma growth factor, and myxoma growth factor) (Prigent and Lemoine 1992; Modjtahedi and Dean 1994). For several of these peptides it has been shown that they can increase tyrosine kinase activity through autocrine, paracrine, intracrine and/or juxtacrine pathways. Furthermore, EGF-like peptides are present in a variety of cell surface and extracellular proteins. The potential function of these peptides as activators of EGFR is of interest, particularly in view of the reports on mitogenic activities of extracellular matrix proteins (Panayotou et al. 1989). The EGF-like growth factor family members are synthesized as transmembrane pre-

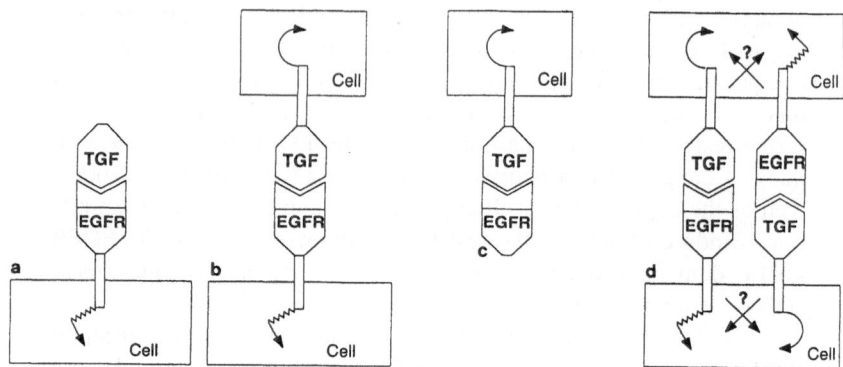

Fig. 1a–d. Bidirectional signaling. **a** Soluble transforming growth factor-α (*TGF*) binds to membrane-anchored receptor. **b** TGF-α and receptor are membrane anchored. **c** Receptor soluble ectodomain binds to membrane-anchored TGF-α. **d** Signal transduction pathways of membrane-anchored partners can cross-modulate. *EGFR*, epidermal growth factor receptor

cursors and specific proteolytic cleavage in the extracellular domain releases the soluble growth factor. A juxtacrine loop can occur when transmembrane growth factors directly activate receptors on the surface of the same cell or immediately adjacent cells (Anklesaria et al. 1990). Recently Shum et al. (1994) demonstrated association of the intracellular part of the TGF-α precursor with a protein kinase complex. This complex displayed activities towards tyrosine, serine, and threonine, suggesting involvement in signal transduction. Thus, if transmembrane TGF-α is involved in "reverse" signal transduction, then it is conceivable that bidirectional communication occurs between adjacent cells following physical interaction of transmembrane TGF-α with its receptor (Fig. 1). These interesting findings by Shum et al (1994) might explain the so far poorly understood presence of secreted extracellular domains of several receptors for growth factors, including EGF/TGF-α, erbB2, nerve growth factor (NGF), interleukin (IL) -2, IL-4, tumor necrosis factor (TNF), and growth hormone. Presumably, secreted extracellular receptor domains may serve as activators for their respective transmembrane ligands. It had been postulated before that the EGF/TGF-α precursors themselves may be receptors, but the experimental evidence had not been presented yet.

Ligands for the EGFR are monomeric in solution and are presumed to bind in a 1:1 stoichiometry. However, the binding of a single EGF molecule to two EGFR in an asymmetrical fashion has also been suggested (Gullick 1994). The structural features of the ligands to the EGFR which comprise three disulfides and, hence, three loops (A, B, and C) have been determined by high-field nuclear magnetic resonance (NMR) studies (Harvey et al 1991; Moy et al. 1993). The consensus of a variety of structural studies on the EGFR ligands is that receptor binding occurs with the involvement of multiple domains. This multidomain-binding model is consistent with the inability of several laboratories to reduce the size of the growth factor without drastically decreasing its affinity for the EGFR. There is no three dimensional structure yet availabile for the EGFR, but there have been NMR studies performed which have examined the binding of TGF-α to a soluble form of the EGFR ectodomain which support the involvement of the A and C loops of TGF-α and the multidomain hypothesis of ligand binding to the EGFR (Hoyt et al. 1994, McInnes et al. 1996).

1.3.2 Dimerization and Receptor Affinity

Two general mechanisms had been suggested to explain the transmembrane signal transduction by EGFR (Ullrich and Schlessinger 1990): (a) EGF binding induces a conformational change of the receptor that propagates through the membrane by a single membrane-spanning domain of EGFR (intramolecular mechanism); (b) EGF binding induces a change in receptor–receptor interaction leading to activation of the cytoplasmic tyrosine kinase (intermolecular mechanism). The intermolecular mechanism was proposed to involve "dimerization and/or microclustering" of EGFR as a necessary prerequisite for the biological response. It has been postulated that inactive receptor monomers are in equilibrium with active receptor dimers and that ligand binding stabilizes the active dimeric or oligomeric form (Lemmon and Schlessinger 1994). An intricate study by Sherill and Kyte (1996) confirmed that activation of EGFR is an equilibrium process. Nevertheless, dimerization of monomeric EGFR did not occur in the absence of bound EGF; dimeric EGFR were only active when two molecules of EGF were bound, and the active complex of EGFR and EGF was equimolar in its stoichiometry. Dimerization can take place between two identical receptors (homodimerization) or between different members of the same receptor family (heterodimerization) (see Sect. 1.5). Ligand binding to EGFR induces heterodimerization of the activated receptor with all three other members of the EGFR family, depending on their numbers and the specific repertoire of a given cell (Earp et al. 1995). The noncovalently associated receptor dimers are considered to represent the high-affinity class of receptors which are active with respect to kinase function. This has been observed with preparations of EGFR homodimers (Böni-Schnetzler and Pilch 1987) as well as with heterodimers of EGFR with erbB2 (Wada et al. 1990; Karunagaran et al. 1996). The high-affinity EGFRs have been proposed to be essential for signal transduction, since their specific inhibition with mAb108 correlated with inhibition of responses to low doses of EGF for all early cellular responses tested (tyrosine-specific phosphorylation of the EGFR, turnover of phosphatidyl inositol, elevation of cytoplasmic pH, and release of Ca^{2+} from intracellular stores; Bellot et al. 1990). High-affinity receptors represent only a minor subclass (1%–10%) of the cell-surface EGFR population and they are preferentially associated to the nondetergent insoluble cytoskeleton as demonstrated using various electron microscopical methods in combination with Scatchard analysis (van Bergen en Henegouwen et al. 1989). The cytoskeleton-associated receptors have been shown to retain a functional ligand-binding domain and EGF-induced kinase activity. Using the specific properties of mAb 2E9, which blocks EGF binding to the low affinity receptor population, while leaving EGF binding to the high-affinity receptors unimpaired, evidence has been provided for a functional difference between low- and high-affinity receptors (Defize et al. 1989). It was demonstrated that activation of the EGFR-mediated signal transduction cascade can occur predominantly through the high-affinity EGFR population, although this population constitutes only a minor proportion of the total receptor population (Defize et al. 1989). It is therefore tempting to suggest that the cytoskeleton-associated EGFR population has a prominent function in signal transduction.

1.3.3 Phosphorylation

Dimerization allows for the so-called receptor autophosphorylation, which represents more an intermolecular cross-phosphorylation of activated kinase domains (Honegger et al. 1990). Phosphorylation of the intracellular EGFR tyrosine residues acts as a molecular switch to create binding sites for cellular proteins containing so-called src homology 2 (SH2) domains. SH2 domains bind specifically to phosphotyrosine residues in the context of a particular amino acid sequence and are responsible for the recruitement of downstream signaling molecules to an activated receptor (Anderson et al. 1990). While some SH2-containing molecules are used as phosphorylation substrates by receptor tyrosine kinases, others are not phosphorylated, but function as adapters to mediate complex formation between receptors and other cellular proteins. This recruitment step constitutes the mechanism of activation of the various cytoplasmic signaling pathways. Furthermore, this domain appears to have a negative regulatory function, as truncation of the carboxy-terminal domain has led to constitutive EGFR activity (Khazaie et al. 1988; Massoglia et al. 1990).

The SH2 domain is a common feature of many nonreceptor kinases which act in the signal cascade downstream of activated growth factor receptors. This is the major structural feature responsible for interaction of phospholipase C (PLC), phosphatidylinositol (PI)3-kinase and ras-GTPase activating protein (GAP) with the activated EGFR (Anderson et al. 1990). Recruitment of these molecules to the cell surface through "docking" with the autophosphorylated EGFR C-terminal tyrosine residues and their subsequent phosphorylation and/or conformational modulation have been proposed to lead to their activation and secondary signal transduction. The affinity of EGFR for these molecules is variable, being high for PLC but particularly low for PI3-kinase. However, there are some reports questioning the stringent requirement of specific autophosphorylation sites for EGFR signaling (Decker 1993; Soler et al. 1994). Receptor activation and function in intact cells does not always seem to require tyrosine autophosphorylation (Lichtner et al. 1992).

Dephosphorylation of autophosphorylated growth factor receptors by protein tyrosine phosphatases (PTPases) appear to represent major mechanisms of negative regulation of tyrosine kinase signaling (Feng et al. 1993; Feng and Pawson 1994). The attenuation of growth factor receptor signaling and reversion of transformation by overexpression of PTPases has been demonstrated (Mooney et al. 1992; Lammers et al. 1993); the SH2 domain containing PTPase, PTP1C, has been shown to associate with the phosphorylated EGF receptor in human tumor cells (Tomic et al. 1995). This interaction between tyrosine kinase receptor and PTPIC is ligand dependent and appears to be positively regulated by phosphatidic acid. Ser/Thr-specific phosphorylation has been observed for a number of PTPases and this may serve to regulate this activity in vivo. Additionally, Ca^{2+}, cAMP, and the ganglioside GM3 have been shown to activate PTPases, though the exact mechanisms are unclear. The regulation of autophosphorylated EGFR by phosphatases is a relatively new area of research but has the potential of uncovering additional targets for therapeutic intervention.

1.3.4 Janus Kinase Signal Transducer and Activator of Transcription

Recently, it has been shown that in addition to the well-characterized Ras mitogen-activated protein kinase signaling pathway ligand-induced activation of the EGFR can trigger the JAK (Janus kinase) STAT (signal transducer and activator of transcription) pathway shared by members of the cytokine receptor superfamily (Silvennoinen et al. 1993; Sadowski et al. 1993). JAKs are nonreceptor tyrosine kinases which associate with the cytokine receptor cytoplasmic tails and upon activation become phosphorylated and initiate subsequent phosphorylation events on a family of proteins known as STATs. The phosphorylated STATs form a complex, become translocated to the nucleus, and activate gene expression by forming specific DNA-binding complexes (Ihle 1996; Ihle et al. 1994). In the case of the EGFR it has been shown the JAK1 and members of the STAT family of transcription factors (STAT1, STAT3, STAT5) are phosphorylated in response to EGF and other ligands (Shuai et al. 1993). Furthermore, it has been shown that the EGFR can directly phosphorylate STATs without the presense of JAK1 (David et al. 1996). This additional signaling pathway utilizing STATs may help to reconcile the variety of cellular responses to EGFR activation. The differential expression of different sets of genes by the EGFR may depend upon the cell-specific availability of certain STATs and the modulation of the Ras-mediated signal.

1.3.5 Cross-Talk

There is increasing evidence that certain growth factors can mediate the action of steroid receptors (Ignar-Trowbridge et al. 1993; McLachlan et al. 1991), notably, the estrogen receptor (ER). It has been demonstrated that EGF and TGF-α can induce ER-dependent transcription of estrogen response elements (ERE) in ER-positive human adenocarcinoma cells expressing the EGFR (Ignar-Trowbridge et al. 1996). Furthermore, a synergistic response to combinations of estrogen and TGF-α or EGF was observed in the activation of transcription. The response elicited by the growth factors alone was independent of PKC and involved a mechanism with distinct features from E_2 mediated ER response. Though the exact mechanism for this receptor cross-talk is not understood, these studies demonstrate that peptide growth factors such as ligands to the EGFR may provide alternative ways of modulating hormonal activity and may represent a general regulatory mechanism for modulating hormonal activity.

Another recent example of cross-talk involves transactivation of receptor tyrosine kinases, such as the EGFR through G-protein-coupled receptor (GPCR) systems. It has been shown that the EGFR becomes rapidly tyrosine-phosphorylated upon stimulation of Rat-1 fibroblast cells with the GPCR agonists, endothelin-1, thrombin, and lyosophatidic acid (Daub et al. 1996). The phosphorylation of EGFR in the system is ligand independent and results in downstream signaling and induction of fos gene expression. These results show that the growth factor mitogens working through the GPCR system can transactivate the EGFR.

1.4 Receptor Mutants

Several reports have documented spontaneous rearrangements within the EGFR gene that arose in primary human glioblastoma tumors (Yamazaki et al. 1988; Ekstrand et al. 1992; Wong et al. 1992). These alterations were always in-frame deletions that preserved the reading frame of the receptor message. The most common of these arrangements was the EGFRvIII, which involves a deletion between nucleotides 275–1075 in the normal EGFR cDNA sequence (Ekstrand et al. 1992; Wong et al. 1992) and is reported to be unique to malignancies (de Palazzo et al. 1993). This mutation generates a fusion junction sequence in the extracellular domain, which is localized outside, but in close proximity to the ligand-binding region. However, as was shown with glioblastoma, expression of the truncated variant gets lost upon primary cell culture (Humphrey et al. 1988) and systems with stable transfection of the gene had to be used. NR6 cells transfected with EGFRvIII expressed membrane-bound, truncated protein with similar autokinase activity as compared with wild-type receptor, but with extremly low affinity for EGF, and hardly any ligand-induced enhancement of receptor phosphorylation. However, the deletion mutant EGFRvIII was capable of transforming immortalized rodent fibroblasts in culture and developing tumors in nude mice independent of ligand (Batra et al. 1995). It has been shown that EGFRvIII can constitutively activate downstream signal transduction through MAP kinase and thus bypass ligand dependence (Montgomery et al. 1995). With the availability of antibodies specific for the mutant protein it could be demonstrated that the variant is more frequently expressed than had been anticipated in primary tumor samples of, for example, non-small-cell lung carcinoma (de Palazzo et al. 1993), breast, ovarian, pediatric glioma, and medulloblastoma tumors (Moscatello et al. 1995). It remains to be seen in larger studies how frequently this variant is expressed and the significance of its contribution to tumor growth and development. However, it may provide a unique and powerful target for a number of forms of cancer detection and treatment.

1.5 The erbB Receptor Family

Three additional transmembrane molecules have considerable sequence homology to the EGFR; however, they differ remarkably in their ligand specificity and kinase function. The four transmembrane tyrosine kinases constitute the type 1 growth factor receptors or erbB receptor family: erbB1 or the EGFR, erbB2, erbB3 and erbB4 (for recent reviews see: Earp et al. 1995; Mason and Gullick 1995). With the exception of betacellulin (Riese et al. 1996), ligands that specifically bind to the EGFR do not directly interact with erbB2, erbB3, or erbB4. Both erbB3 and erbB4 bind all isoforms of an EGF-related factor called Neu differentiation factor (NDF, or heregulin). ErbB2 binds no known ligand, but its catalytic action is relatively high and it seems to have an inherent propensity to dimerize with itself when it is overexpressed. This is in strong contrast to EGFR, which despite overexpression does not signal without ligand. These four receptors are shown to form heterodimers in a ligand-dependent manner, and these may even form when only one member of the pair binds its ligand. The formation of heterodimers occurs preferentially to homodimers and these complexes have a higher kinase activity than the respective homodimers. ErbB3 is an especially intriguing molecule, since it is thought to have very low intrinsic kinase activity. However, in cells expressing erbB2 and erbB3 tyrosine phosphorylation of both receptors was found upon heregulin addition. Since heregulin cannot bind to erbB2 alone, erbB3 must provide the initial binding site and a cooperative interaction with erbB2 must then result in high-affinity complexes. Furthermore, since erbB3 lacks an intrinsic kinase activity, it is not clear how heregulin can promote the tyrosine phosphorylation of erbB2. This finding is in contrast to the concept of tyrosine phosphorylation occurring via transphosphorylation of receptors within a dimeric complex (see Sect. 1.3.2). Heterodimerization of EGFR with any other member of the family is strictly ligand dependent. In EGFR/erbB2 heterodimers the affinity for EGF was increased (Wada et al. 1990), apparently due to deceleration of ligand dissociation rates (Karunagaran et al. 1996). It has been suggested that the transphosphorylation of heterologous receptors within a ligand-induced dimer serves to modulate the growth regulatory signal by determining which SH2 domain containing intracellular signaling proteins are recruited to the activated receptor complex (Carraway and Cantley 1994). While EGFR and erbB2 appear to bind to a broadly similar set of second messenger molecules (for review see: Mason and Gullick 1995), erbB3 seems to signal via PI3-kinase, whereas EGFR and erbB2 only form very weak complexes with this molecule (Fedi et al. 1994).

Thus, when compared to ligand-dependent receptor homodimers comprised of two proteins with the same internalization sequence and phosphorylated tyrosine residues, heterodimers are likely to (a) expand substrate selection and downstream signaling pathway activation, (b) promote interaction between sets of substrates in the mixed receptor complexes that would not normally be physically juxtaposed, (c) alter the duration of receptor signaling by changing rates of receptor internalization, ligand loss, kinase inactivation, recycling, and (d) alter rates of receptor and substrate dephosphorylation. It is now apparent that the ability of EGFR and the other members of the family to form heterodimers can increase the number of possible signaling active dimers in a combinatorial fashion, thus increasing the diversity and control of cellular signals.

1.6 Summary

The significance of EGFR for embryonal development and epithelial cell differentiation has been demonstrated by using EGFR knockout and TGF-α transgenic mice. EGFR activity has been shown to initiate or contribute to progression of neoplasia in a wide range of experimental systems. In various human epithelial malignancies, expression of EGFR is associated with poor prognosis. In such carcinomas, paracrine, autocrine or juxtacrine activation of EGFR seems to be a common means of promoting growth and/or dissemination. Truncations or mutations of EGFR may contribute to aberrant EGFR signaling in human tumors. Ligand-induced heterodimerization of EGFR with other members of the family can increase the number of possible signaling active dimers in a combinatorial fashion, thus increasing the diversity and control of cellular signals.

Acknowledgments. We would like to acknowledge Dr. Stewart Thompson and Dr. Kashayarsha Khazaie for helpful discussions.

References

Anderson D, Koch CA, Grey L, Ellis C, Moran MF, Pawson T (1990) Binding of SH2 domains of phospholipase C1, GAP, and src to activated growth factor receptors. Science 250: 979–982

Anklesaria P, Teixidó J, Laiho M, Pierce JH, Greenberger JS, Massagué J (1990) Cell-cell adhesion mediated by binding of membrane-anchored transforming growth factor to epidermal growth factor receptors promotes cell proliferation. Proc Natl Acad Sci USA 87: 3289–3293

Batra SK, Castelino-Prabhu S, Wikstrand CJ, Zhu X, Humphrey PA, Friedman HS, Bigner DD (1995) Epidermal growth factor ligand-independent, unregulated, cell-transforming potential of a naturally occurring human mutant EGFRvIII gene. Cell Growth Differ 6: 1251–1259

Bellot F, Moolenar W, Kris R, Mirakhur B, Verlaan I, Ullrich A, Schlessinger J, Felder S (1990) High-affinity epidermal growth factor binding is specifically reduced by a monoclonal antibody, and appears necessary for early responses. J Cell Biol 110: 491–502

Böni-Schnetzler M, Pilch PF (1987) Mechanism of epidermal growth factor receptor autophosphorylation and high-affinity binding. Proc Natl Acad Sci USA 84: 7832–7835

Carraway III KL, Cantley LC (1994) A neu acquaintance for erbB3 and erbB4: a role for receptor heterodimerization in growth signaling. Cell 78: 5–8

Daub, H , Weiss FU , Wallasch C, Ullrich A (1996) Role of transactivation of the EGF receptor in signalling by G-protein-coupled receptors. Nature 379:557–564.

David M, Wong L, Flavell R, Thompson SA, Wells A, Larner AC, Johnson GR (1996) STAT activation by epidermal growth factor (EGF) and amphiregulin. J Biol Chem 271:9185–9188 .

Decker SJ (1993) Transmembrane signaling by epidermal growth factor receptors lacking autophosphorylation sites. J Biol Chem 268:9176–9179

Defize LHK, Boonstra J, Meisenhelder J, Kruijer W, Tertoolen LGJ, Tilly BC, Hunter T, van Bergen en Henegouwen PMP, Moolenar WH, de Laat SW (1989) Signal transduction by epidermal growth factor occurs through the subclass of high affinity receptors. J Cell Biol 109: 2495–2507

de Palazzo IEG, Adams GP, Sundaseshan P, Wong AJ, Testa JR, Bigner DD, Weiner LM. (1993) Expression of mutated epidermal growth factor receptor by non-small cell lung carcinoma. Cancer Res 53: 3217–3220

Earp HS, Dawson TL, Li X, Yu H (1995) Heterodimerization and functional interaction between EGF receptor family members: a new signaling paradigm with implications for breast cancer research. Breast Cancer Res Treat 35: 115–132

Ekstrand AJ, Sugawa N, James CD, Collins VP (1992) Amplified and rearranged epidermal growth factor receptor genes in human glioblastomas reveal deletions of sequences encoding portions of the N- and/or C-terminal tails. Proc Natl Acad Sci USA 89: 4309–4313

Fedi P, Pierce JH, Difiore PP, Kraus MH (1994) Efficient coupling with phosphatidylinositol 3-kinase, but not phospholipase c- or GTPase-activating protein, distinguishes erbB-3 signaling from that of other erbB-EGFR family members. Mol Cell Biol 14: 492–500

Feng GS, Pawson T (1994) Phosphotyrosine phosphatases with SH2 domains: regulators of signal transduction. Trends Genet 10:54–58.

Feng GS, Hui CC, Pawson T (1993) SH2-containing phosphotyrosine phosphatase as a target of protein-tyrosine kinases. Science 259:1607–1611

Gullick WJ (1991) Prevalence of aberrant expression of the epidermal growth-factor receptor in human cancers. Br Med Bull 47:87–98

Gullick WJ (1994) A new model for the interaction of EGF-like ligands with their receptors: the new one-two. Eur J Cancer 30: 2186–2188

Harvey TS, Wilkinson AJ, Tappin MJ, Cooke RM, Campbell ID (1991) The solution structure of human transforming growth factor α. Eur J Biochem 198: 555–562

Honegger AM, Schmidt A, Ullrich A, Schlessinger J (1990) Evidence for epidermal growth factor receptor-induced intermolecular autophosphorylation of the EGF-receptors in living cells. Mol Cell Biol 10:4035–4044

Hoyt DW, Harkins RN, Debanne MT, O'Connor-McCourt M, Sykes BD (1994) Interaction of transforming growth factor α with the epidermal growth factor receptor: finding kinetics and differential mobility within the bound TGF-α. Biochemistry 33:15283–15292

Humphrey PA, Wong AJ, Vogelstein B, Friedman HS, Werner MH, Bigner DD, Bigner SH (1988) Amplification and expression of the epidermal growth-factor receptor gene in human glioma xenografts. Cancer Res 48: 2231–2238

Hynes NE (1993) Amplification and overexpression of the c-erbB-2 gene in human tumors: its involvement in tumor development, its significance as a prognostic factor, and its potential as a target for cancer therapy. Semin Cancer Biol 4:19–26

Ignar-Trowbridge DM, Teng CT, Ross KA, Parker Mg, Korach KS, McLachlan JA (1993) Peptide growth factors elicit estrogen receptor dependent transcriptional activation of an estrogen-responsive element. Mol Endocrinol 7:992–998

Ignar-Trowbridge DM, Pimantel M, Parker MG, McLachlan JA, Korach KS (1996) Peptide growth factor cross-talk with the estrogen receptor requires the A/B domain and occurs independently of protein kinase C or estradiol. Endocrinology 137:1735–1744

Ihle JN (1996) STATs: signal transducers and activators of transcription. Cell 84:331–334

Ihle JN, Witthuhn BA, Quelle FW, Yamamoto K, Thierfelder WE, Kreider B, Silvennoinen O (1994) Signaling by the cytokine receptor superfamily: JAKs and STATs. Trends Bioch Sci 19:222–227

Jhappan C, Stahle C, Harkins RN, Fausto N, Smith GH, Merlino GT (1990) TGF-α overexpression in transgenic mice induces liver neoplasia and abnormal development of the mammary gland and pancreas. Cell 61: 1137–1146

Karunagaran D, Tzahar E, Beerli RB, Chen X, Graus-Porta D, Ratzkin BJ, Seger R, Hynes NE, Yarden Y (1996) ErbB-2 is a common auxiliary subunit of NDF and EGF receptors: implications for breast cancer. EMBO J 15:254–264

Khazaie K, Dull TJ, Graf T, Schlessinger J, Ullrich A, Beug H, Vennström B (1988) Truncation of the human EGFR leads to differential transforming potentials in primary avian fibroblasts and erythroblasts. EMBO J 7:3061–3071

Lammers R, Bossenmaier B, Cool DE, Tonks K, Schlessinger J, Fischer EH, Ullrich A (1993) Differential activities of protein tyrosine phosphatases in intact cells. J Biol Chem 268:22456–22462

Lemmon MA, Schlessinger J (1994) Regulation of signal transduction and signal diversity by receptor oligomerization. Trends Biochem Sci 19: 459–463

Lichtner RB, Wiedemuth M, Kittmann A, Ullrich A, Schirrmacher V, Khazaie K (1992) Ligand-induced activation of epidermal growth factor receptor in intact rat mammary adenocarcinoma cells without detectable receptor phosphorylation. J Biol Chem 267:11872–11880

Mason S, Gullick WJ (1995) Type 1 growth factor receptors: an overview of recent developments. Breast 4: 11–18

Massoglia S, Gray A, Dull TJ, Munemitsu S, Kung H-J, Schlessinger J, Ullrich A (1990) Epidermal growth factor receptor cytoplasmic domain mutations trigger ligand-independent transformation. Mol Cell Biol 10:3048–3055

McInnes C, Hoyt DW, Harkins RH, Debanne MT, O'Connor-McCourt M, Sykes BD (1996) NMR study of the transforming growth factor alpha/epidermal growth factor receptor complex: visualization of ligand binding determinants through NOE analysis of free and bound hTGFα. Biochemistry (in press)

McLachlan JA, Nelson KG, Takahashi T, Bossert NL, Newborn RR, Korach KS (1991) Estrogens and growth factors in the development, growth, and function of the female reproductive tract. Schomberg DW (ed) Growth factors in reproduction. Springer, New York, pp 197–203

Miettinen PJ, Berger JE, Meneses J, Phung Y, Pederson RA, Werb Z, Derynck R (1995) Epithelial immaturity and multiorgan failure in mice lacking epidermal growth factor receptor. Nature 376: 337–341

Modjtahedi H, Dean C (1994) The receptor for EGF and its ligands: expression prognostic value and target for therapy in cancer. Int J Oncol 4:277–296

Montgomery RB, Moscatello DK, Wong AJ, Cooper JA, Stahl WL (1995) Differential modulation of mitogen-activated protein (MAP) kinase/extracellular signal-related kinase kinase and MAP kinase activities by a mutant epidermal growth factor receptor. J Biol Chem 270: 30562–30566

Mooney RA, Freund GG, Way BA, Bordell KL (1992) Expression of a transmembrane phosphotyrosine phosphatase inhibits cellular response to platelet-derived growth factor and insulin-like growth factor. J Biol Chem 267:23443–23446

Moscatello DK, Holgado-Madruga M, Godwin AK, Ramirez G, Gunn G, Zoltick PW, Biegel JA, Hayes RL, Wong AJ (1995) Frequent expression of a mutant epidermal growth factor receptor in multiple human tumors. Cancer Res 55:5536–5539

Moy FJ, Li Y-C, Ravenbuehler P, Winkler ME, Scheraga HA, Montelione GT (1993) Solution structure of human type-α transforming growth factor determined by heteronuclear NMR spectroscopy and refined by energy minimization with restraints. Biochemistry 32:7334–7353

Nicholson S, Halcrow P Jr, Sainsbury C, Angus B, Chambers P, Farnon JR, Harris AL (1988) Epidermal growth factor receptor (EGFR) status associated with failure of primary endocrine therapy in elderly postmenopausal patients with breast cancer. Br J Cancer 58:810–814

Panayotou G, End P, Aumailley M, Timpl R, Engel H (1989) Domains of laminin with growth factor activity. Cell 56: 93–101

Prigent SA, Lemoine NR (1992) The type1 (EGFR-related) family of growth factor receptors and their ligands. Prog Growth Factor Res 4:1–24

Riese DJ, Bermingham Y, van Raaij TM, Buckley S, Plowman GD, Stern DF (1996) Betacellulin activates the epidermal growth factor receptor and erbB-4, and induces cellular response patterns distinct from those stimulated by epidermal growth factor or neuregulin. Oncogene 12: 345–353

Sadowski HB, Shuai K, Darnell JE, Gilman MZ (1993) A common nuclear signal transduction pathway activated by growth factor and cytokine receptors. Science 261:1739–1742

Sainsbury JRC, Farnon JR, Needham GK, Malcolm AJ, Harris AL (1987) Epidermal-growth factor receptor states as predictor of early recurrence of and death from breast cancer. Lancet i: 1398–1402

Sandgreen EP, Luettke NC, Palmiter RD, Brinster RL, Lee DC (1990) Overexpression of TGF-α in transgenic mice: induction of epithelial hyperplasia, pancreatic metaplasia, and carcinoma of the breast. Cell 61: 1121–1135

Sherill JM, Kyte J (1996) Activation of epidermal growth factor receptor by epidermal growth factor. Biochemistry 35: 5705–5718

Shuai K, Ziemiecki A, Wilks AF, Harpur AG, Sadowski HB, Gilman MZ, Darnell JE (1993) Polypeptide signalling to the nucleus through tyrosine phosphorylation of Jak and Stat proteins. Nature 366:580–582

Shum L, Reeves SA, Kuo AC, Fromer ES, Derynck R (1994) Association of the transmembrane TGF-α precursor with a protein kinase complex. J Cell Biol 125: 903–916

Sibilia M, Wagner EF (1995) Strain-dependent epithelial defects in mice lacking the EGF receptor. Science 269: 234–238

Silvennoinen O, Schindler C, Schlessinger J, Levy DE (1993) Ras-independent growth factor signaling by transcription factor tyrosine phosphorylation. Science 261:1736–1739

Slamon DJ, Clark GM, Wong SG, Levin WJ, Ullrich A, McGuire WL (1987) Human breast cancer: correlation of relapse and survival with amplification of the HER-2/neu oncogene. Science 235:177–182

Soler C, Beguinot L, Carpenter G (1994) Individual epidermal growth factor receptor autophosphorylation sites do not stringently define association motifs for several SH2-containing proteins. J Biol Chem 269: 12320–12324

Threadgill DW, Dlugosz AA, Hansen LA, Tennenbaum T, Lichti U, Yee D, LaMantia C, Mourton T, Herrup K, Harris RC, Barnard JA, Yuspa SH, Coffey RJ, Magnuson T (1995) Targeted disruption of mouse EGF receptor: effect of genetic background on mutant phenotype. Science 269:230–234

Tomic S, Greiser U, Lammers R, Kharitonenkov A, Imyanitov E, Ullrich A, Böhmer F-D (1995) Association of SH2 domain protein tyrosine phosphatases with the epidermal growth factor receptor in human tumor cells. J Biol Chem 270:21277–21284

Ullrich A, Schlessinger J (1990) Signal transduction by receptors with tyrosine kinase activity. Cell 61: 203–212

van Bergen en Henegouwen PMP, Defize LHK, de Kroon J, van Damme H, Verkleij AJ, Boonstra J (1989) Ligand-induced association of epidermal growth factor receptor to the cytoskeleton of A431 cells. J Cell Biochem 39:455–465

Wada T, Qian X, Greene MI (1990) Intermolecular association of the p185[neu] protein and EGF receptor modulates EGF receptor function. Cell 61: 1339–1347

Wong AJ, Ruppert JM, Bigner SH, Grzeschik CH, Humphrey PA, Bigner DS, Vogelstein B (1992) Structural alterations of the epidermal growth factor gene in human gliomas. Proc Natl Acad Sci USA 89: 2965–2969

Yamazaki H, Fukui Y, Ueyama Y, Tamaoki N, Kawamoto T, Taniguchi S, Shibuya M (1988) Amplification of the structurally and functionally altered epidermal growth factor receptor gene (c-erbB) in human brain tumors. Mol Cell Biol 8: 1816–1820

2 Characterization of Growth Factor Receptor-Directed Protein Tyrosine Phosphatases

F.-D. Böhmer

2.1 Introduction

Dimerization of growth factor receptor tyrosine kinases (RTK) (Heldin 1995) leads in turn to a mutual phosphorylation of two receptor monomers at multiple tyrosine residues. This process, commonly designated as "autophosphorylation" is the initial and a crucial event of growth factor signaling, which is followed by initiation of a multitude of downstream signaling chains (Ullrich and Schlessinger 1990; Fantl et al. 1993). RTK autophosphorylation serves two purposes: (1) It regulates the activity of the RTK positively, albeit to a different extent for different receptor species. Determination of the three-dimensional structure of the catalytic center of the insulin receptor has recently shed some light on the structural basis for the pronounced activation of this RTK by autophosphorylation (Hubbard et al. 1994). Tyrosine 1162 in the un-phosphorylated form sterically blocks access to the peptide substrate and the ATP binding sites. In the phosphorylated form it is expected to become disengaged from the active center and to allow access of the substrates. In terms of homology it is possible that such a mechanism might operate similarly in other RTK. (2) Autophosphorylation creates binding sites for intracellular proteins possessing phosphotyrosine binding domains such as SH2 or PTB domains (Pawson 1995). Although some aspects of receptor signaling seem to be retained in autophosphorylation-impaired RTK mutants (Decker 1993; N.X. Li et al. 1994; Blakesley et al. 1995) and even signaling of kinase-inactive RTK has been reported (Coker et al. 1994), it has been clearly shown for many RTK that defined signaling chains cannot be initiated in the absence of the respective phosphotyrosine docking site for a certain downstream signaling molecule. For example, elimination of binding sites for phospholipase Cγ on the platelet-derived growth factor (PDGF) receptor (tyrosine 1009 and 1021) (Rönnstrand et al. 1992) abrogates PDGF-stimulated activation of phosphoinositide hydrolysis (Valius et al. 1993). Thus, regulation of receptor autophosphorylation deserves much attention. Evidence is mounting that in addition to ligand binding, RTK autophosphorylation is tightly controlled by several intracellular mechanisms. One of these mechanisms is the dephosphorylation of autophosphorylated receptors by protein-tyrosine phosphatases (PTPases). Concomitant with the discovery of RTK activity, the existence of such potent enzymes was observed. It took, however, until 1989 to structurally identify the first PTPase – PTP1B (Charbonneau et al. 1989). Since then, many and structurally very diverse PTPases have been discovered and characterized in much detail (Charbonneau and Tonks 1992; Barford et al. 1995; Dixon 1995). Functional data linking members of the large PTPase family to the phenomenon of RTK dephosphorylation are, however, relatively rare. We have attempted to characterize PTPases involved in dephosphorylation of autophosphorylated epidermal growth factor (EGF) and PDGF receptors. Starting from the investigation of special characteristics of receptor dephosphorylation we are trying to identify involved PTPase molecules. This approach might complement the more common strategy to look for physiological substrates of previously identified PTPases.

2.2 Characterization of Receptor-Directed PTPases in Swiss 3T3 Cell Membranes

To obtain more information on the characteristics of the RTK dephosphorylation phenomenon we have compared parameters of dephosphorylation of two RTK, EGF RTK and PDGF RTK, which are expressed at similar levels in Swiss 3T3 cells. Both receptors transmit mitogenic signals in these cells. Plasma membranes were isolated and receptor dephosphorylation parameters were estimated subsequently to stimulation of the RTK with the cognate ligand, autophosphorylation in the presence of $[\gamma^{32}P]ATP$ and quenching of the kinase reaction either by addition of a large excess of unlabeled ATP, depletion of ATP by an ATP-consuming reaction or by complexing the manganese essential for the kinase reaction with ethylene diamine tetraacetate (EDTA). The receptor dephosphorylation kinetics were strikingly different (Böhmer et al. 1993). EGF receptors were much faster dephosphorylated at all temperatures tested than PDGF receptors. This observation, which later was confirmed by similar data obtained in intact cells (see below), might relate to the known difference in mitogenic potency of EGF and PDGF in these cells: PDGF elicits a more sustained mitogenic response than EGF. Very rapid EGF receptor dephosphorylation we also observed in A431 cell membranes, human placenta membranes (F.D.Böhmer, S.A.Böhmer, and C.H.Heldin, unpublished), and in EGF receptor overexpressing 293 cells (T. Echternacht, F.D. Böhmer, unpublished). Another interesting observation was made when the pH profiles for the receptor dephosphorylation rate were determined (Böhmer et al. 1993). While both receptors reveal little difference, the rate is optimal between pH 6 and 7 and drops sharply towards more alkaline pH values. Almost no dephosphorylation of EGF receptor can be seen above pH 8. Thus, subtle changes in intracellular pH might affect signaling via the receptor dephosphorylation rate. One might speculate that the known alkalinization of the cell interior upon mitogenic stimulation contributes to the generation of the mitogenic signal by attenuating PTPase reaction. When different agents known to have effects on isolated PTPases were tested for their effect on RTK dephosphorylation, surprisingly, sodium orthovanadate was only partially inhibitory, whereas zinc acetate potently inhibited receptor dephosphorylation (Table 1). The EGF receptor

Table 1. Effect of various compounds on receptor dephosphorylation in Swiss 3T3 cell membranes. (Modified from Böhmer et al. 1993)

Compound	Concentration	Relative dephosphorylating activity (% of control)	
		EGFR	PDGFR
Vanadate	0.01 mM	84	67
	0.1 mM	76	69
	1 mM	67	76
Zn acetate	0.01 mM	80	84
	0.1 mM	16	27
	1 mM	0	6
Spermine	2 mM	99	78
Protamine	25 µg/ml	83	19
Poly-lysine	25 µg/ml	95	46
Triton X-100	1%	49	74
Octylglucoside	1%	46	70

EGFR, epidermal growth factor receptor; PDGFR, platelet-derived growth factor receptor.

and PDGF receptor-directed PTPase(s) differed with respect to their sensitivity to some agents, exemplified by polyamines and detergents. While PDGF receptor dephosphorylation was strongly blocked by protamine and polylysine, EGF receptor dephosphorylation was refractory to these agents. In contrast, EGF receptor dephosphorylation was more strongly impaired by detergents (Table 1; Böhmer et al. 1993). The differential sensitivity of EGF and PDGF receptor dephosphorylation to various agents suggests the involvement of different PTPase species in both cases.

We also investigated the possible effect of growth state or heterologous growth factor stimulation on RTK dephosphorylation in isolated Swiss 3T3 cell membranes (F.D.Böhmer, S.A.Böhmer, unpublished). To this end, large-scale cell cultures of Swiss 3T3 cells were subjected to growth factor treatment or were harvested at different cell densities. Then, membranes were isolated and receptor dephosphorylation kinetics were measured as described. Whereas no effect of cell density was observed in these experiments on dephosphorylation of either RTK, a finding later confirmed for intact cells (see below), growth factor stimulation with either PDGF or the equally potent combination of EGF and

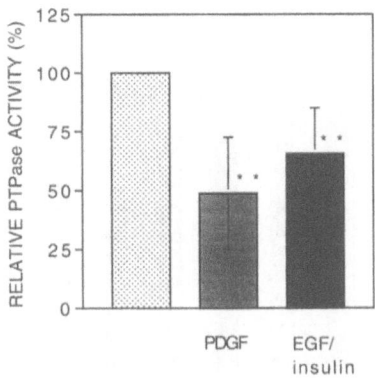

Fig. 1. Effect of growth factor treatment of Swiss 3T3 cells on the epidermal growth factor (*EGF*) receptor dephosphorylation rate in subsequently isolated cell membranes. Confluent Swiss 3T3 cell cultures were treated in serum-free medium with platelet-derived growth factor (*PDGF,* 10 ng/ml) or the combination of EGF (10 ng/ml) and insulin (1 µg/ml) or were left untreated for 2 h, as indicated. Then, cell membranes were isolated and the relative dephosphorylation rate of autophosphorylated EGF receptor was determined. Means ± SD of six independent experiments are depicted. ** *p<0.01 for comparison with membranes from untreated cells*

insulin led to a reduced EGF receptor dephosphorylation rate in the subsequently isolated membranes (Fig. 1). These findings define another level of putative receptor cross-talk. A synergistic activity of growth factors could be related to negative mutual effects on receptor dephosphorylation. Intact cell experiments are, however, required to further substantiate such a hypothesis.

An interesting subject is the specificity of receptor dephosphorylation with respect to certain phosphorylation sites. Concluding from experiments with synthetic phosphopeptides (Cho et al. 1993; Milarski et al. 1993; Sugimoto et al. 1993; Zhang et al. 1994), preference of certain PTPases for individual phosphorylation sites is likely. While no in vivo data are yet available in this respect, recent in vitro experiments by Klinghoffer and Kazlauskas (Klinghoffer and Kazlauskas 1995) seem to support the concept of site-specific RTK dephosphorylation. When autophosphorylated PDGF receptor was exposed to the action of PTPases PTP1D or PTP1B, clear differences in dephosphorylation ki-

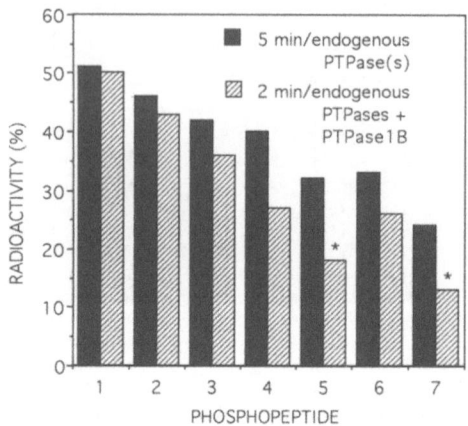

Fig. 2. Differences in autophosphorylation site specificity between endogenous platelet-derived growth factor (PDGF) receptor-directed PTPases in Swiss 3T3 cell membranes and PTP1B. PDGF receptor was stimulated and allowed to autophosphorylate in the presence of $[\gamma^{32}P]ATP$. The phosphorylation was quenched by addition of ethylene diamine tetraacetate and dephosphorylation was allowed for the indicated times at 25°C in the presence of 5 mM dithiothreitol (DTT) and in the absence or presence of 1 µg/ml of human recombinant PTPase 1B, as indicated. The samples were separated by sodium dodecyl sulfate polyacrylamide gel electrophoresis and gel sections containing the autophosphorylated receptor were extracted. The extracts were digested with trypsin and the obtained phosphopeptides were separated on 40% acrylamide gels in the presence of urea. The dried gels were analyzed with a Phosphorimager to quantitate the relative radioactivity in seven phosphopeptides *P1–P7* generated from PDGF receptor. The relative content of radioactivity in the individual peptides (the value obtained at 0 min was set 100%) obtained from PDGF receptor when dephosphorylated for 5 min in the absence or for 2 min in the presence of PTPase 1B is compared. Under these conditions, an enhanced dephosphorylation of peptides P5 and P7 in the presence of PTPase 1B (*) was observed in multiple independent experiments

netics of the different sites were observed. Such "fingerprinting" might help to identify the responsible PTPases in vivo, although in the intact cell protection of phosphorylation sites by bound SH2 domain proteins is likely to affect the dephosphorylation patterns (Rotin et al. 1992; Lammers et al. 1993). We analyzed dephosphorylation kinetics of EGF or PDGF receptors in Swiss 3T3 cell membranes at the level of tryptic phosphopeptides (F.D. Böhmer, S.A. Böhmer, C.H.Heldin, E. Hoppe, A. Ullrich, unpublished). The radioactive receptor bands corresponding to different time points of dephosphorylation were extracted and subjected to tryptic digestion and one-dimensional dense-gel separation. In case of EGF receptor, these peptides are representative of single phosphorylation sites. We observed a similar rate of dephosphorylation of all EGF receptor peptides by the endogenous PTPase(s). Addition of recombinant PTPase 1B accelerated dephosphorylation of all peptides to a similar extent (not shown). In case of the PDGF receptor, addition of PTPase 1B also accelerated dephosphorylation of all peptides (not shown); however, compared to the action of the endogenous PTPase(s) alone, a preference of PTPase 1B for certain peptides was observed. This becomes obvious by comparing the relative radioactivity in the different PDGF receptor peptides in a typical experiment, as shown in Fig. 2. After 5 min of receptor dephosphorylation in the absence of PTPase 1B and after 2 min dephosphorylation in the presence of PTPase 1B, peptides P1, P2, P3, and P6 contained similar amounts of radioactivity under both conditions. Peptides P5 and P7, however, contained in the presence of PTPase 1B clearly less radioactivity than in its absence. Thus, PTP1B seems to have a substrate specificity which is different from that of the endogenous PTPases. These experiments and other considerations make it unlikely that PTP1B contributes to PDGF receptor dephosphorylation in Swiss 3T3 cells. Extension of site-specific dephosphorylation experiments to intact cells will be informative not only with respect to the possibly involved PTPases but will have also implications for understanding receptor autophosphorylation dynamics as a result of combined RTK and PTPase action and reveal possible selective PTPase effects on some signaling pathways, but not others.

2.3 Lipid Modulation of EGF Receptor-Directed PTPase(s)

As described above and also found by others, detergents inhibit EGF receptor dephosphorylation in membranes. This effect suggests the possible importance of the lipid environment for the PTPase-RTK interaction. Also, lipid effects on the activity of isolated PTPases have been described (Zhao et al. 1993, 1994). We therefore tested the effect of various lipids on EGF receptor dephosphorylation in A431 cell mem-

Table 2. Effect of different lipids on EGFR dephosphorylation rate

Lipid	Effect at concentration	
	50 µg/ml	100 µg/ml
Phosphatidic acid	+	+
Lysophosphatidic acid	0	−
Phosphatidylserine	−	−
Phosphatidylinositol	−	−
Cardiolipin	0	(+)
Phosphatidylethanolamine	0	(+)
Diacylglycerol	0	0
Sphingomyelin	0	0
Arachidonic acid	0	0
Oleic acid	0	0
Palmitic acid	0	0

The various lipids at the indicated concentrations were added to A431 cell membranes. Then, the resident EGF receptors were stimulated, and allowed to autophosphorylate in the presence of $[\gamma^{32}P]ATP$. The kinase reaction was quenched by addition of ethylene diamine tetraacetate and dephosphorylation rates were estimated by sodium dodecyl sulfate polyacrylamide gel electrophoresis and Phosphorimage analysis at different time points.
0, no effect; +, acceleration; −, inhibition; EGFR, epidermal growth factor receptor.

branes (Table 2). Whereas most lipids had little effect in these assays, phosphatidic acid activated receptor dephosphorylation. In contrast, lysophosphatidic acid and phophatidylserine inhibited the dephosphorylation reaction (U.Greiser and F.D. Böhmer, unpublished). Activation of EGF receptor dephosphorylation by phosphatidic acid was later also seen in other systems and helped to identify PTP1C as one of the PTPases contributing to EGF receptor dephosphorylation (see below).

Another lipid modulation of EGF receptor dephosphorylation we came across when we investigated the cytostatic effects of ganglioside GM3 on an EGF receptor expressing NSCLC line, NCI H125 (E. Suarez Pestana, U. Greiser, B. Sanchez, L.E.Fernandez, A. Lage, R. Perez, F.D. Böhmer, submitted). The growth of this cell line is driven at least in part by an autocrine activation of resident EGF receptors. Treatment of the cells with anti-EGF receptors antibodies, with specific EGF RTK inhibi-

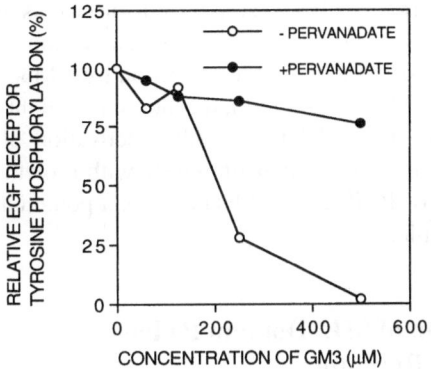

Fig. 3. Effect of ganglioside GM3 treatment on epidermal growth factor (EGF) receptor phosphorylation in NCI H125 non-small-cell lung carcinoma cells. Subconfluent cultures of H125 cells were treated with ganglioside GM3 at the indicated concentrations for 2 h in serum-free medium. Thereafter, the cells were stimulated with EGF, extracted and the EGF receptor phosphorylation was analyzed by sodium dodecyl sulfate polyacrylamide gel electrophoresis and immunoblotting with anti-phosphotyrosine antibodies. In one series (indicated), the cells were in addition treated with 100 μ*M* pervanadate for 30 min before EGF stimulation, whereas control cells were treated with the respective solvent (vehicle). Phosphorylation of the EGF receptor was quantitated by densitometry and relative values, compared to not GM3 treated cells (100%) are depicted

tors, or with ganglioside GM3 blocked EGF receptor autophosphorylation as well as cell growth. When the GM3 treatment was performed in the presence of the PTPase inhibitor pervanadate, no inhibition of EGF receptor autophosphorylation by GM3 could be observed anymore, suggesting that the GM3 effect is mediated by a PTPase rather than a direct effect on the RTK (Fig. 3). Similar observations were made when A431 epidermoid carcinoma cells were subjected to GM3 treatment. These findings prompted us to directly measure the possible effect of GM3 on the EGF receptor dephosphorylation rate in A431 cell membranes. Indeed, GM3 pretreatment of the membranes clearly accelerated EGF receptor dephosphorylation. Since in contrast to phosphatidic acid, GM3 is unlikely to enter the cells one could speculate that an interaction with transmembrane PTPases at the cell surface is involved in the activation. We are currently trying to test various transmembrane PTPases with respect to a possible activation by GM3. Similarly to the study of phosphatidic acid (below), this approach might help to identify an EGF receptor-directed PTPase. Also, activation of EGF receptor dephosphorylation by GM3 concomitantly with growth inhibition suggests activation of RTK-directed PTPases as a potentially useful novel cytostatic principle.

2.4 Interaction of SH2-Domain PTPases with the EGF Receptor

One obvious approach to identify RTK-directed PTPases seems to be to search for RTK-associated PTPase molecules. To this end, we isolated the EGF receptor from A431 cell membrane preparations (Tomic et al. 1995). Indeed, PTPase-activity towards an exogenous synthetic substrate – [^{32}P]Raytide – was found in the receptor isolates and clearly copurified with the receptor in several steps of chromatography. The PTPase activity could partly be displaced from the receptor by treatment with phenylphosphate, suggesting the involvement of SH2 domains in the PTPase-EGF receptor interaction. We, therefore, investigated the possible presence of the two hitherto known SH2-domain PTPases – PTP1C (SH-PTP1, SHC, HCP) or PTP1D (SH-PTP2, syp, SH-PTP3, PTP2C) (see Feng and Pawson 1994, for review) – in the receptor preparations. Both PTPases were detectable. Further evidence for an association of both PTPases with the EGF receptor could be obtained by co-immunoprecipitation experiments using intact A431 cells (Fig. 4). The latter experiments also revealed that the association, although detectable in non-EGF-stimulated cells, is strongly enhanced by EGF stimulation. When we subjected the EGF receptor preparation isolated along with the PTPases to dephosphorylation experiments, we observed to our surprise rather little activity of the associated PTPases towards the receptor (Fig. 5A). We speculated that this might be a consequence of the isolation in the presence of detergents and possible depletion of important lipids. Therefore, different lipids were tested for possible restoration of PTPase activity towards the EGF receptor. Phosphatidic acid, which we had found before to activate EGF receptor dephosphory-

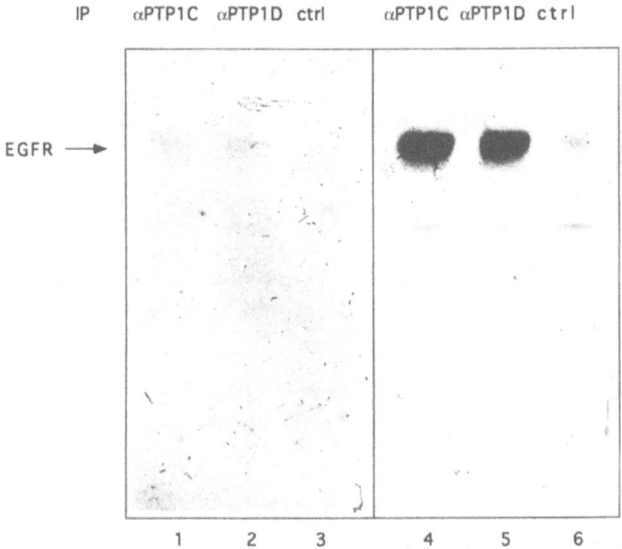

Fig. 4. Detection of epidermal growth factor receptor (*EGFR*) in anti-PTP1C and anti-PTP1D immunoprecipitates. Serum-deprived sub-confluent cultures of A431 cells were left unstimulated (*lanes 1–3*) or were stimulated with 100 ng/ml EGF for 10 min at room temperature (*lanes 4–6*). Cell lysates were prepared and subjected to immunoprecipitation with anti-PTP1C antibodies (*lanes 1, 4*), anti-PTP1D antibodies (*lanes 2, 5*) or non-specific IgG (*lanes 3, 6*). Subsequently, the samples were incubated on ice in the presence of [γ^{32}P]ATP and manganese to allow autophosphorylation and then subjected to sodium dodecyl sulfate polyacrylamide gel electrophoresis and autoradiography (from Tomic et al. 1995 with permission of the publisher)

lation in A431 cell membranes (see above), increased EGF receptor-directed PTPase activity in the receptor isolates significantly (Fig. 5B). This finding supported our hypothesis that the receptor-associated SH2-domain PTPases might be involved in receptor dephosphorylation in the intact cell. Indeed, when intact A431 cells were treated with phosphatidic acid, we found that the level of EGF receptor autophosphorylation was reduced. The effect of phosphatidic acid was abrogated by pretreatment of the cells with pervanadate, suggesting the involvement of PTPases in the reduction of EGF receptor phosphorylation level (Tomic

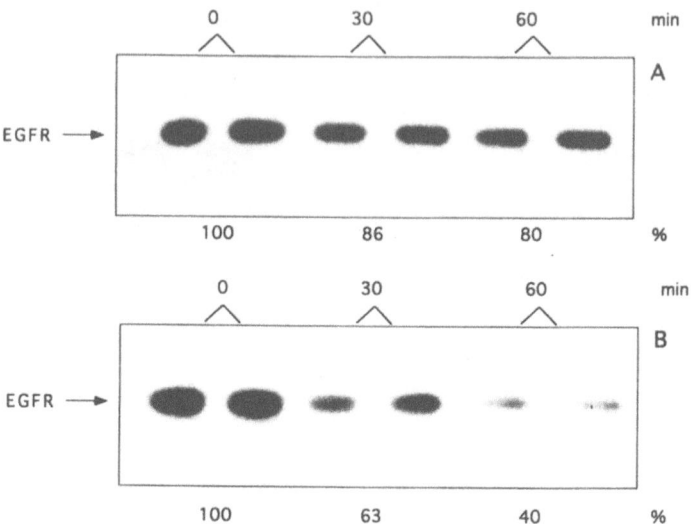

Fig. 5A,B. Phosphatidic acid activates epidermal growth factor receptor (*EGFR*) dephosphorylation by the receptor-associated PTPase(s). Column-purified EGF receptor was incubated in the absence (**A**) or presence of 50 µg/ml phosphatidic acid (**B**) for 20 min on ice. Then, the receptor was allowed to autophosphorylate in the presence of [γ^{32}P]ATP, the phosphorylation was quenched by addition of EDTA, the samples were transferred to 37°C and the radioactivity in the receptor was monitored at the indicated time-points by sodium dodecyl sulfate polyacrylamide gel electrophoresis and autoradiography. *Numbers* underneath the *lanes* represent the percentage of radioactivity (mean of the duplicates, 100% at time-point 0 min) as obtained by densitometric quantification (from Tomic et al. 1995, with permission of the publisher)

et al. 1995). To further investigate whether PTP1C or PTP1D or both would mediate the phosphatidic acid effect, the two PTPases were transiently coexpressed with the EGF receptor in 293 cells. As observed earlier by Vogel et al. (Vogel et al. 1993), PTP1C coexpression clearly reduced the EGF receptor phosphorylation level in this system, whereas PTP1D was without effect. Phosphatidic acid had little influence in case of PTP1D and EGF receptor coexpression but strongly enhanced the PTP1C effect. Taking these data together, we propose that PTP1C contributes to EGF receptor dephosphorylation in intact cells with phosphatidic acid being a putative positive regulator. Such a role of phosphatidic

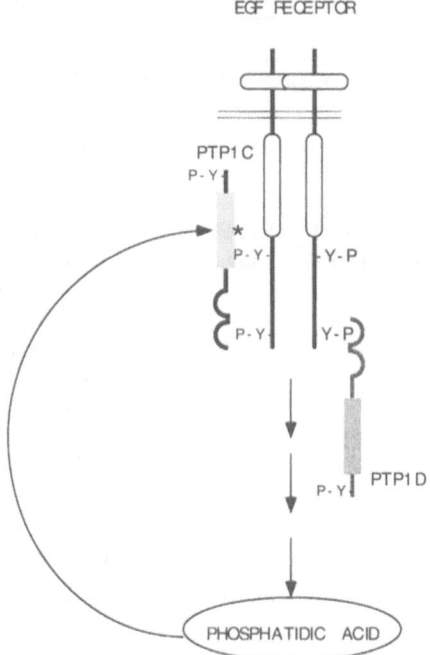

Fig. 6. Hypothetical negative feed-back regulation of epidermal growth factor (*EGF*) receptor signaling by phosphatidic acid. Schematic illustration of EGF receptor signaling which leads over several steps to an increase of phosphatidic acid levels in A431 cells. Phosphatidic acid has the potency to activate EGF receptor-directed activity of PTP1C, but has no activity on the likewise EGF receptor-associated PTPase PTP1D. *P-Y*, phosphotyrosine; *activity of PTPIC towards the receptor

acid might make sense as part of a negative feedback regulation for EGF receptor signaling activity since EGF treatment has been shown to increase phosphatidic acid levels in A431 cells drastically (Fig. 6).

PTP1C has by now been implicated in negative regulation of several RTK (see Table 3). In addition, evidence for a negative role of PTP1C for signaling of cytokine receptors (Yi et al. 1993; Klingmuller et al. 1995), B-cell antigen receptors (Cyster and Goodnow 1995; Pani et al. 1995), and the FcγIIB1 receptor (D'Ambrosio et al. 1995) has been

Table 3. PTPases possibly involved in negative regulation of certain RTK

RTK	PTPase species	References
Insulin receptor	RPTPα, LAR, PTP1C, CD45	Hashimoto et al. 1992; Vogel et al. 1993; Møller et al. 1995; Kulas et al. 1995, 1996a,b; Ahmad et al. 1995
PDGF receptor	CD45, LAR, RPTPα, PTP1D, PTP1C, low M_r PTP	Mooney et al. 1992; Vogel et al. 1993; Lammers et al. 1993; Berti et al. 1994; Klinghoffer and Kazlauskas 1995
EGF receptor	PTP1C, LAR, RPTPσ	Vogel et al. 1993; Tomic et al. 1995; Kulas et al. 1996a; Aicher 1996
Kit/SCF receptor	PTP1C, PTP1D, CD45	Yi and Ihle 1993; Vogel et al. 1993; Lammers et al. 1993

RTK, receptor tyrosine kinase; PDGF, platelet-derived growth factor; EGF, epidermal growth factor.

obtained. Thus PTP1C seems capable for interaction with a wide range of receptors, leading to attenuation of signaling activity. In contrast, PTP1D seems not to participate in RTK dephosphorylation, with the possible exception of Kit/SCF receptor (Vogel et al. 1993) and PDGF receptor (Klinghoffer and Kazlauskas 1995). Instead, evidence is mounting for a positive role of PTP1D in mediation of RTK signals, although the substrates for the PTPase in such a process are still elusive. The question arises as to which structural properties of the two rather homologous SH2-domain PTPases lead to the strikingly different inter-action with RTK. One structural determinant might be the specificity of the SH2 domains. One could envisage that differential positioning of the PTPases by their SH2 domains on the autophosphorylated receptor would allow dephosphorylation of neighboring phosphotyrosines in case of PTP1C and not in case of PTP1D. On the other hand, the catalytic domain specificity could permit PTP1C but not PTP1D to

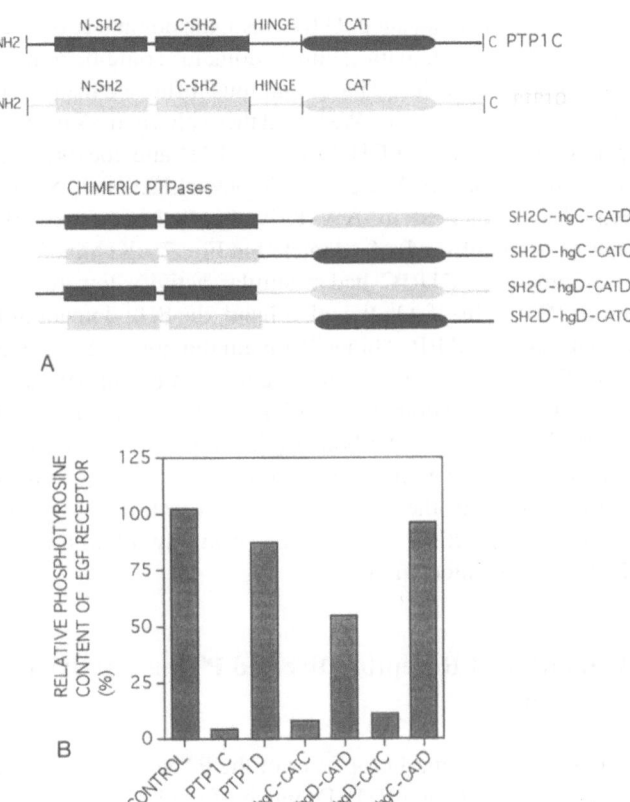

Fig. 7A,B. Interaction of chimerical PTPases derived from PTP1C and PTP1D with the epidermal growth factor (EGF) receptor in 293 cells. **A** Schematic illustration and designation of different chimerical PTPases generated from PTP1C and PTP1D by domain "swapping". **B** Effect of coexpression of various PTPase derivatives with the EGF receptor in 293 cells on receptor tyrosine phosphate content. Some 293 cells were transfected with EGF receptor alone (control) or in combination with the depicted PTPases. Cell lysates were analyzed for EGF receptor tyrosine phosphorylation by immunoblotting with anti-phosphotyrosine antibodies. Quantitation of a representative immunoblot is shown. EGF receptor expression and PTPase expression was comparable in all variants

dephosphorylate the associated RTKs. Also, the domain in between SH2 domains and catalytic domain ("hinge" domain) could be important for the overall structure of the PTPases and thus influence the activity with respect to the associated RTK. We tested these alternatives by generating different chimeras between PTP1C and PTP1D and coexpressing them with the EGF receptor in 293 cells (T.Tenev, H.Keilhack, S. Tomic, B. Stoyanov, M. Gerlach-Stein, A.V. Krivtsov, R. Lammers, A. Ullrich, F.D. Böhmer, unpublished). As depicted in Fig. 7, all chimeras with the catalytic domain of PTP1C had a similar activity towards the EGF receptor as PTP1C itself. On the other hand, the SH2 domain of PTP1C with or without the PTP1C "hinge" domain did not confer activity with respect to EGF receptor dephosphorylation to the catalytic domain of PTP1D. Thus, the SH2 domain specificity seems of little importance for the differential activity of the both PTPases towards the EGF receptor and rather the catalytic domain specificity seems crucial. Further dissection of the latter with the same "swap" approach might yield further insights into the structural basis for the strikingly differential SH2-domain PTPase-RTK interaction.

2.5 Regulation of Receptor-Directed PTPase Activity in Intact Cells

In addition to the structural properties of the PTPase as discussed above for the case of PTP1C and PTP1D, much of the specificity of PTPase-RTK interaction in the intact cell might be brought about by cellular localization (Mauro and Dixon 1994) and by regulation of PTPase activity via different mechanisms (Table 4). Thus, studying PTPase RTK interaction in vitro or in isolated membranes, which may be informative, might not reveal important features of receptor dephosphorylation. Therefore, it seems desirable to measure RTK dephosphorylation directly in intact cells. When both PTPase and RTK are highly overexpressed in recipient cells as 293 cells, judgment of the activity of the overexpressed PTPase is easily obtained by evaluation of the receptor phosphotyrosine content in the absence or the presence of the PTPase (Lammers et al. 1993). If RTK–PTPase interaction is to be analyzed at more physiological levels, it is difficult to differentiate with this technique between effects of a certain cell manipulation on either

Table 4. Mechanisms possibly involved in regulation of cellular PTPase activity

Process	PTPase	References
Serine/threonine-specific phosphorylation	RPTPα	DenHertog et al. 1995
	PTP1B	Flint et al. 1993; Schievella et al. 1993
	PTP1C, PTP1D	Zhao et al. 1994; Peraldi et al. 1994; Trachman et al. 1995
	PTP-PEST	Garton and Tonks 1994
	CD45	Stover and Walsh 1994
Tyrosine phosphorylation	PTP1D	Vogel et al. 1993; Zhao et al. 1994; Feng et al. 1993; W. Li et al. 1994
	PTP1C	Uchida et al. 1994; Bouchard et al. 1994
	RPTPα	DenHertog et al. 1994; Su et al. 1994
Dimerization	CD45	Desai et al. 1993
Occupation of SH2 domains	PTP1D	Lechleider et al. 1993
	PTP1C	Pei et al. 1994
Lipid interaction	PTP1C, PTP1D	Zhao et al. 1993, 1994
Partial proteolysis	T-cell PTP	Cool et al. 1990
	PTP1D	Zhao et al. 1994
Homophilic interactions of extracellular domains	PTPμ, PTPκ	Gebbink et al. 1993; Brady-Kalnay et al. 1993; Brady-Kalnay and Tonks 1994; Sap et al. 1994
Shedding of extracellular domain	LAR, RPTPσ	Serra-Pages et al. 1994; Aicher 1996
Binding of extracellular ligands	RPTPβ	Peles et al. 1995
Expression level	LAR	Longo et al. 1993
	DEP1	Östman et al. 1994
	RPTPσ	Celler et al. 1995

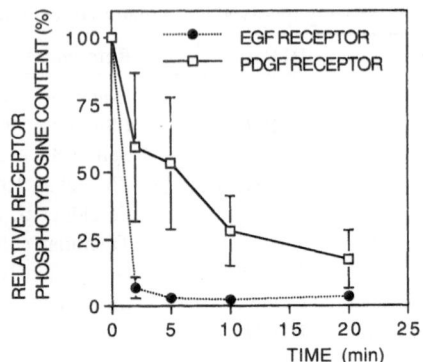

Fig. 8. Time course of platelet-derived growth factor (*PDGF*) receptor and epidermal growth factor (*EGF*) receptor dephosphorylation in Swiss 3T3 cells. Quiescent Swiss 3T3 cells were treated with EGF or with PDGF for 5 min at room temperature. Then, the specific tyrosine kinase blockers AG1517 or AG1296, respectively, were added and the phosphotyrosine content of the receptors was analyzed by sodium dodecyl sulfate polyacrylamide gel electrophoresis and immunoblotting at different time points. Means of three independent experiments are shown. (From Böhmer et al. 1995 with permission of the publisher)

the RTK activity or on the PTPase activity. To overcome this problem, quenching of the RTK activity and subsequent monitoring of the decay of receptor phosphotyrosine content has been employed. A problem with this method exists in that the hitherto used quenching agents such as EDTA are not readily cell permeable. Cell permeabilization has, therefore, to be applied using these agents, which might in turn destroy important regulatory interactions. We therefore wondered whether potent and selective tyrosine kinase inhibitors which became available recently (Kovalenko et al. 1994; Levitzki and Gazit 1995) might serve as more suitable agents to quench the RTK activity. To serve such a purpose, the respective compounds should rapidly enter the cells and inhibit the RTK but have no effect on the RTK-directed PTPases. We found that the tyrphostins AG1296, AG1517 and the staurosporine derivative K252a fulfill these criteria and are useful tools to measure PTPase activity in intact cells directed against PDGF receptor, EGF receptor, and NGF receptor (TrkA), respectively (Böhmer et al. 1995).

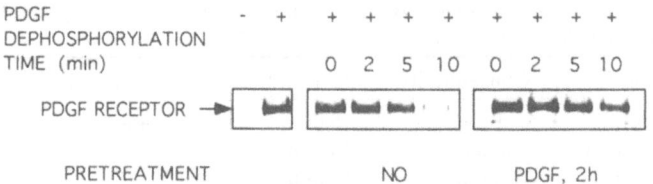

Fig. 9. Effect of platelet-derived growth factor (*PDGF*) pretreatment on PDGF receptor dephosphorylation in Swiss 3T3 cells. Quiescent Swiss 3T3 cells were treated in the absence or presence of 10 ng/ml PDGF for 2 h in serum-free medium, as indicated. Then, the cells were stimulated with 100 ng/ml PDGF for 5 min, the PDGF receptor blocker AG1296 was added and subsequently the PDGF receptor dephosphorylation was monitored by immunoblotting

When we used this method to investigate RTK dephosphorylation in intact Swiss 3T3 cells, several interesting observations were made. As found earlier in cell membrane experiments (see above), EGF and PDGF receptors are dephosphorylated with remarkably different kinetics (Fig. 8). EGF receptor dephosphorylation proceeds very rapidly, while the PDGF receptors are dephosphorylated to only 50% within 2–5 min. PDGF receptor dephosphorylation was investigated more closely for effects of cell growth conditions or cell treatments which we suspected to be important for regulation of receptor-directed PTPase activity. In agreement with our data in isolated cell membranes, no effect on receptor dephosphorylation was observed when 3T3 cells at different culture densities were investigated (Böhmer et al. 1995). PDGF treatment of the cells, however, reduced the receptor dephosphorylation rate significantly (Fig. 9). Such treatment was found previously (Celler et al. 1995) to reduce expression of a transmembrane PTPase in Swiss 3T3 cells – mRPTPα – and one might speculate that both events are linked. We are currently testing the possible role of RPTPα for PDGF receptor dephosphorylation.

Ser/Thr-specific phosphorylation has been observed for a number of PTPase species (Table 4) and suggested to regulate activity in the intact cell. When we tested the effect of known modulators of Ser/Thr-kinases on PDGF receptor-directed PTPase activity in Swiss 3T3 cells, we found significant activation of this process by elevators of Ca^{2+} and

Table 5. Activation of PDGF receptor dephosphorylation in intact Swiss 3T3 cells by elevators of intracellular Ca2+ and cAMP

Effector	Concentration	Time of treatment	Effect plus-minus
A23187	1 μM	5 min	+++
Thapsigargin	30 nM	30 min	+
Forskolin	100 μM	15 min	+
IBMX	5 mM	1 h	++
AlF3	10 mM	1 h	++

Confluent Swiss 3T3 cells were treated with the listed reagents at the indicated concentrations for the indicated time at 37°C in serum-free medium. Then, plate-derived growth factor receptor dephosphorylation rate was measured. Control, 100% relative PTPase activity; +, 100–150%; ++, 150–200%; +++, 200–250%.

cAMP (Table 5) (F.D.Böhmer and S.A. Böhmer, submitted). These findings are in agreement with the concept that PDGF receptor-directed PTPases can be activated by Ca^{2+} and cAMP-dependent protein kinases, although other more indirect mechanisms cannot be excluded at present. Again, the observed characteristics of PDGF receptor-directed PTPase(s) will hopefully aid in identifying the enzymes involved among the many candidates.

2.6 Summary and Perspectives

Dephosphorylation of EGF RTK is very rapid and seems to affect all autophosphorylation sites similarly. Both SH2-domain PTPases, PTP1C and PTP1D, are capable of interacting with EGF receptors; however, only PTP1C seems to be involved in dephosphorylation of the RTK, a property not related to different SH2-domain specificity but rather to a different catalytic domain specificity of the two related PTPases. Phosphatidic acid activates PTP1C with respect to its activity towards the EGF receptor and might present part of a negative feedback loop for regulation of EGF RTK signaling activity. Ganglioside GM3 likewise activates EGF receptor dephosphorylation via activation of an as yet unknown PTPase. At the same time GM3 inhibits EGF receptor-driven growth of human non-small-cell lung carcinoma cells.

PDGF receptor dephosphorylation is comparatively slow and not affected by cell density in Swiss 3T3 cells. It is inhibited by PDGF treatment and activated by elevation of Ca2+ and cAMP levels. Indirect data suggest the possible involvement of RPTPα in PDGF receptor dephosphorylation.

Future work will aim at identifying more of the PTPases involved in EGF and PDGF receptor dephosphorylation, assuming that several enzyme species will be involved in this process. Application of known characteristics with respect to regulation of RTK dephosphorylation, the use of permanent cell lines with an increased and, in particular, decreased expression level of certain candidate PTPases, and possibly "fingerprinting" of autophosphorylation-site specific dephosphorylation will be important tools towards this goal.

Our data show clearly that receptor-directed PTPase activity is subject to regulation by extracellular stimuli and therefore presents an interesting novel target for cytostatic or cytotrophic agents.

References

Ahmad F, Considine RV, Goldstein BJ (1995) Increased abundance of the receptor-type protein-tyrosine phosphatase LAR accounts for the elevated insulin receptor dephosphorylating activity in adipose tissue of obese human subjects. J Clin Invest 95:2806–2812

Aicher B (1996) Untersuchungen zur Spezifität und Regulation der Phosphotyrosinphosphatasen LAR und PTPσ. Thesis. University of Munich

Barford D, Jia ZC, Tonks NK (1995) Protein-tyrosine phosphatases take-off. Nat Struct Biol 2:1043–1053

Berti A, Rigacci S, Raugei G, Deglinnocenti D, Ramponi G (1994) Inhibition of cellular response to platelet-derived growth factor by low M(r) phosphotyrosine protein phosphatase overexpression. FEBS Lett 349:7–12

Blakesley VA, Kato H, Roberts CT, Leroith D (1995) Mutation of a conserved amino acid residue (tryptophan 1173) in the tyrosine kinase domain of the IGF-I receptor abolishes autophosphorylation but does not eliminate biologic function. J Biol Chem 270:2764–2769

Böhmer FD, Böhmer SA, Heldin CH (1993) The dephosphorylation characteristics of the receptors for epidermal growth factor and platelet-derived growth factor in Swiss 3T3-cell membranes suggest differential regulation of receptor signalling by endogenous protein-tyrosine phosphatases. FEBS Lett 331:276–280

Böhmer FD, Böhmer A, Obermeier A, Ullrich A (1995) Use of selective tyrosine kinase blockers to monitor growth-factor receptor dephosphorylation in intact-cells. Anal Biochem 228:267–273

Bouchard P, Zhao ZZ, Banville D, Dumas F, Fischer EH, Shen SH (1994) Phosphorylation and identification of a major tyrosine phosphorylation site in protein tyrosine phosphatase 1C. J Biol Chem 269:19585–19589

Brady-Kalnay SM, Tonks NK (1994) Identification of the homophilic binding site of the receptor protein tyrosine phosphatase PTP μ. J Biol Chem 269:28472–28477

Brady-Kalnay SM, Flint AJ, Tonks NK (1993) Homophilic binding of PTP-μ, a receptor-type protein tyrosine phosphatase, can mediate cell cell aggregation. J Cell Biol 122:961–972

Celler JW, Luo XM, Gonez LJ, Böhmer FD (1995) mRNA expression of two transmembrane protein tyrosine phosphatases is modulated by growth factors and growth arrest in 3T3 fibroblasts. Biochem Biophys Res Commun 209:614–621

Charbonneau H, Tonks NK (1992) 1002 phosphatases? Annu Rev Cell Biol 8:463–493

Charbonneau H, Tonks NK, Kumar S, Diltz CD, Harrylock M, Cool DE, Krebs EG, Fischer EH, Walsh KA (1989) Human placenta protein-tyrosine-phosphatase: amino acid sequence and relationship to a family of receptor-like proteins. Proc Natl Acad Sci USA 86:5252–5256

Cho H, Krishnaraj R, Itoh M, Kitas E, Bannwarth W, Saito H, Walsh CT (1993) Substrate specificities of catalytic fragments of protein tyrosine phosphatases (HPTP beta, LAR, and CD45) toward phosphotyrosylpeptide substrates and thiophosphotyrosylated peptides as inhibitors. Protein Sci 2:977–984

Cool DE, Tonks NK, Charbonneau H, Fischer EH, Krebs EG (1990) Expression of a human T-cell protein-tyrosine-phosphatase in baby hamster kidney cells. Proc Natl Acad Sci USA 87:7280–7284

Cyster JG, Goodnow CC (1995) Protein tyrosine phosphatase 1C negatively regulates antigen receptor signaling in B lymphocytes and determines thresholds for negative selection. Immunity 2:13–24

D'Ambrosio D, Hippen KL, Minskoff SA, Mellman I, Pani G, Siminovitch KA, Cambier JC (1995) Recruitment and activation of PTP1C in negative regulation of antigen receptor signaling by Fc gamma RIIB1. Science 268:293–297

Decker SJ (1993) Transmembrane signaling by epidermal growth factor receptors lacking autophosphorylation sites. J Biol Chem 268:9176–9179

DenHertog J, Tracy S, Hunter T (1994) Phosphorylation of receptor protein-tyrosine phosphatase alpha on Tyr789, a binding site for the SH3-SH2-SH3 adaptor protein GRB-2 in vivo. EMBO J 13:3020–3032

DenHertog J, Sap J, Pals C, Schlessinger J, Kruijer W (1995) Stimulation of receptor protein-tyrosine phosphatase alpha activity and phosphorylation by phorbol ester. Cell Growth Differ 6:303–307

Desai DM, Sap J, Schlessinger J, Weiss A (1993) Ligand-mediated negative regulation of a chimeric transmembrane receptor tyrosine phosphatase. Cell 73:541–554

Dixon JE (1995) Structure and catalytic properties of protein-tyrosine phosphatases. Ann N Y Acad Sci 766:18–22

Fantl WJ, Johnson DE, Williams LT (1993) Signalling by receptor tyrosine kinases. Annu Rev Biochem 62:453–481

Feng GS, Pawson T (1994) Phosphotyrosine phosphatases with Sh2 domains – regulators of signal transduction. Trends Genet 10:54–58

Feng GS, Hui CC, Pawson T (1993) SH2-containing phosphotyrosine phosphatase as a target of protein-tyrosine kinases. Science 259:1607–1611

Flint AJ, Gebbink MF, Franza BJ, Hill DE, Tonks NK (1993) Multi-site phosphorylation of the protein tyrosine phosphatase, PTP1B: identification of cell cycle regulated and phorbol ester stimulated sites of phosphorylation. EMBO J 12:1937–1946

Garton AJ, Tonks NK (1994) PTP-PEST: a protein tyrosine phosphatase regulated by serine phosphorylation. EMBO J 13:3763–3771

Gebbink MFBG, Zondag GCM, Wubbolts RW, Beijersbergen RL, Vanetten I, Moolenaar WH (1993) Cell-cell adhesion mediated by a receptor-like protein tyrosine phosphatase. J Biol Chem 268:16101–16104

Hashimoto N, Feener EP, Zhang WR, Goldstein BJ (1992) Insulin receptor protein-tyrosine phosphatases – leukocyte common antigen-related rhosphatase rapidly deactivates the insulin receptor kinase by preferential dephosphorylation of the receptor regulatory domain. J Biol Chem 267:13811–13814

Heldin CH (1995) Dimerization of cell surface receptors in signal transduction. Cell 80:213–223

Hubbard SR, Wei L, Elis L, Hendrickson WA (1994) Crystal structure of the tyrosine kinase domain of the human insulin receptor. Nature 372:746–754

Klinghoffer RA, Kazlauskas A (1995) Identification of a putative Syp substrate, the PDGF beta receptor. J Biol Chem 270:22208–22217

Klingmuller U, Lorenz U, Cantley LC, Neel BG, Lodish HF (1995) Specific recruitment of SH-PTP1 to the erythropoietin receptor causes inactivation of JAK2 and termination of proliferative signals. Cell 80:72–738

Kovalenko M, Gazit A, Böhmer A, Rorsman C, Ronnstrand L, Heldin CH, Waltenberger J, Böhmer FD, Levitzki A (1994) Selective platelet-derived growth factor receptor kinase blockers reverse sis-transformation. Cancer Res 54:6106–6114

Kulas DT, Zhang WR, Goldstein BJ, Furlanetto RW, Mooney RA (1995) Insulin receptor signaling is augmented by antisense inhibition of the protein tyrosine phosphatase LAR. J Biol Chem 270:2435–2438

Kulas DT, Freund GG, Mooney RA (1996a) The transmembrane protein-tyrosine-phosphatase cd45 is associated with decreased insulin-receptor signaling. J Biol Chem 271:755–760

Kulas DT, Goldstein BJ, Mooney RA (1996b) The transmembrane protein-tyrosine-phosphatase lar modulates signaling by multiple receptor tyrosine kinases. J Biol Chem 271:748–754

Lammers R, Bossenmaier B, Cool DE, Tonks NK, Schlessinger J, Fischer EH, Ullrich A (1993) Differential activities of protein tyrosine phosphatases in intact cells. J Biol Chem 268:22456–22462

Lechleider RJ, Sugimoto S, Bennett AM, Kashishian AS, Cooper JA, Shoelson SE, Walsh CT, Neel BG (1993) Activation of the SH2-containing phosphotyrosine phosphatase SH-PTP2 by its binding site, phosphotyrosine-1009, on the human platelet-derived growth factor receptor-beta. J Biol Chem 268:21478–21481

Levitzki A, Gazit A (1995) Tyrosine kinase inhibition: an approach to drug development. Science 267:1782–1788

Li NX, Schlessinger J, Margolis B (1994) Autophosphorylation mutants of the EGF-receptor signal through auxiliary mechanisms involving SH2 domain proteins. Oncogene 9:3457–3465

Li W, Nishimura R, Kashishian A, Batzer AG, Kim WJH, Cooper JA, Schlessinger J (1994) A new function for a phosphotyrosine phosphatase – linking Grb2-SOS to a receptor tyrosine kinase. Mol Cell Biol 14:509–517

Longo FM, Martignetti JA, Lebeau JM, Zhang JS, Barnes JP, Brosius J (1993) Leukocyte common antigen-related receptor-linked tyrosine phosphatase – regulation of messenger RNA expression. J Biol Chem 268:26503–26511

Mauro LJ, Dixon JE (1994) Zip codes direct intracellular protein tyrosine phosphatases to the correct cellular address. Trends Biochem Sci 19:151–155

Milarski KL, Zhu GC, Pearl CG, McNamara DJ, Dobrusin EM, Maclean D, Thiemesefler A, Zhang ZY, Sawyer T, Decker SJ, Dixon JE, Saltiel AR (1993) Sequence specificity in recognition of the epidermal growth factor receptor by protein tyrosine phosphatase-1B. J Biol Chem 268:23634–23639

Møller N, Møller K, Lammers R, Kharitonenkov A, Hoppe E, Wiberg F, Sures I, Ullrich A (1995) Selective down-regulation of the insulin receptor signal by protein-tyrosine phosphatases alpha, epsilon. J Biol Chem 270:23126–23131

Mooney RA, Freund GG, Way BA, Bordwell KL (1992) Expression of a transmembrane phospotyrosine phosphatase inhibits cellular response to platelet-derived growth factor and insulin-like growth factor. J Biol Chem 267:23443–23446

Östman A, Yang Q, Tonks NK (1994) Expression of DEP-1, a receptor-like protein-tyrosine-phosphatase, is enhanced with increasing cell density. Proc Natl Acad Sci USA 91:9680–9684

Pani G, Kozlowski M, Cambier JC, Mills GB, Siminovitch KA (1995) Identification of the tyrosine phosphatase ptp1c as a b cell antigen receptor-associated protein involved in the regulation of b cell signaling. J Exp Med 181:2077–2084

Pawson T (1995) Protein modules and signalling networks. Nature 373:573–580

Pei DH, Lorenz U, Klingmuller U, Neel BG, Walsh CT (1994) Intramolecular regulation of protein tyrosine phosphatase SH-PTP1: a new function for Src homology 2 domains. Biochemistry 33:15483–15493

Peles E, Nativ M, Campbell PL, Sakurai T, Martinez R, Lev S, Clary DO, Schilling J, Barnea G, Plowman GD, Grumet M, Schlessinger J (1995) The carbonic anhydrase domain of receptor tyrosine phosphatase beta is a functional ligand for the axonal cell recognition molecule contactin. Cell 82:251–260

Peraldi P, Zhao ZH, Filloux C, Fischer EH, Vanobberghen E. (1994) Protein-tyrosine-phosphatase 2C is phosphorylated and inhibited by 44-kDa mitogen-activated protein kinase. Proc Natl Acad Sci USA 91:5002–5006

Rönnstrand L, Mori S, Arridsson AK, Eriksson A, Wernstedt C, Hellman U, Claessonwelsh L, Heldin CH (1992) Identification of 2 C-terminal autophosphorylation sites in the PDGF beta-receptor – involvement in the interaction with phospholipase-C-gamma. EMBO J 11:3911–3919

Rotin D, Margolis B, Mohammadi M, Daly RJ, Daum G, Li N, Fischer EH, Burgess WH, Ullrich A, Schlessinger J (1992) SH2 domains prevent tyrosine dephosphorylation of the EGF receptor: identification of Tyr992 as the high-affinity binding site for SH2 domains of phospholipase Cγ. EMBO J 11:559–567

Sap J, Jiang YP, Friedlander D, Grumet M, Schlessinger J (1994) Receptor tyrosine phosphatase R-Ptp-kappa mediates homophilic binding. Mol Cell Biol 14:1–9

Schievella AR, Paige LA, Johnson KA, Hill DE, Erikson RL (1993) Protein tyrosine phosphatase-1B undergoes mitosis-specific phosphorylation on serine. Cell Growth Differ 4:239–246

Serra-Pages C, Saito H, Streuli M (1994) Mutational analysis of proprotein processing, subunit association, and shedding of the LAR transmembrane protein tyrosine phosphatase. J Biol Chem 269:23632–23641

Stover DR, Walsh KA (1994) Protein-tyrosine phosphatase activity of CD45 is activated by sequential phosphorylation by two kinases. Mol Cell Biol 14:5523–5532

Su J, Batzer A, Sap J (1994) Receptor tyrosine phosphatase R-PTP-alpha is tyrosine-phosphorylated and associated with the adaptor protein Grb2. J Biol Chem 269:18731–18734

Sugimoto S, Lechleider RJ, Shoelson SE, Neel BG, Walsh CT (1993) Expression, purification, and characterization of SH2-containing protein tyrosine phosphatase, SH-PTP2. J Biol Chem 268:22771–22776

Tomic S, Greiser U, Lammers R, Kharitonenkov A, Imyanitov E, Ullrich A, Böhmer FD (1995) Association of SH2 domain protein tyrosine phosphatases with the epidermal growth factor receptor in human tumor cells. Phosphatidic acid activates receptor dephosphorylation by PTP1C. J Biol Chem 270:21277–21284

Trachman JD, Huang J, Reem GH (1995) Activation of human thymocytes induces the phosphorylation of protein tyrosine phosphatase 1C. C R Acad Sci III 318:367–374

Uchida T, Matozaki T, Noguchi T, Yamao T, Horita K, Suzuki T, Fujioka Y, Sakamoto C, Kasuga M (1994) Insulin stimulates the phosphorylation of Tyr(538) and the catalytic activity of Ptp1C, a protein tyrosine phosphatase with SRC homology-2 domains. J Biol Chem 269:12220–12228

Ullrich A, Schlessinger J (1990) Signal transduction by receptors with tyrosine kinase activity. Cell 61:203–212

Valius M, Bazenet C, Kazlauskas A (1993) Tyrosines 1021 and 1009 are phosphorylation sites in the carboxy terminus of the platelet-derived growth factor receptor beta subunit and are required for binding of phospholipase C gamma and a 64-kilodalton protein, respectively. Mol Cell Biol 13:133–143

Vogel W, Lammers R, Huang J, Ullrich A (1993) Activation of a phosphotyrosine phosphatase by tyrosine phosphorylation. Science 259:1611–1614

Yi T, Ihle JN (1993) Association of hematopoietic cell phosphatase with c-Kit after stimulation with c-Kit ligand. Mol Cell Biol 13:3350–3358

Yi TL, Mui ALF, Krystal G, Ihle JN (1993) Hematopoietic cell phosphatase associates with the interleukin-3 (IL-3) receptor-beta chain and down-regulates IL-3-induced tyrosine rhosphorylation and mitogenesis. Mol Cell Biol 13:7577–7586

Zhang ZY, Maclean D, McNamara DJ, Sawyer TK, Dixon JE (1994) Protein tyrosine phosphatase substrate specificity – size and phosphotyrosine positioning requirements in peptide substrates. Biochemistry 33:2285–2290

Zhao ZH, Shen SH, Fischer EH (1993) Stimulation by phospholipids of a protein-tyrosine-phosphatase containing 2 src homology-2 domains. Proc Natl Acad Sci USA 90:4251–4255

Zhao ZZ, Larocque R, Ho WT, Fischer EH, Shen SH (1994) Purification and characterization of Ptp2C, a widely distributed protein tyrosine phosphatase containing two Sh2 domains. J Biol Chem 269:8780–8785

3 Interaction of Heparin-Binding EGF-Like Growth Factor with Multiple Receptors

K. Elenius, G. Allison, S.K. Das, B.C. Paria, S.K. Dey, and M. Klagsbrun

3.1 Introduction

Heparin-binding epidermal growth factor-like growth factor (HB-EGF) was first characterized as a heparin-binding mitogen secreted by cultured human macrophages (Besner et al. 1990) and subsequently cloned and sequenced from the human macrophage-like cell line U-937 (Higashiyama et al. 1991). HB-EGF was considered to be a member of the family of EGF-like growth factors based on its primary structure containing six conserved cysteine residues (Higashiyama et al. 1992) and on its ability to compete for the binding of ^{125}I-labeled EGF to the surfaces of A431 cells overexpressing EGF receptor (EGFR; Higashiyama et al. 1991). Similar properties are shared by other members of the family, including EGF itself (Savage et al. 1972; Cohen et al. 1980), transforming growth factor-α (TGF-α) (Derynck et al. 1984), amphiregulin (Shoyab et al. 1989), schwannoma-derived growth factor (Kimura et al. 1990), betacellulin (Shing et al. 1993) and epiregulin (Toyoda et al. 1995). In addition to these "classical" members of the family, several groups have independently reported the purification of a gene product that has a domain homologous to the six cysteine structure of EGF but that cannot directly bind EGFR. This factor is expressed in several alternatively spliced forms and has been named heregulin (Holmes et al. 1992), Neu differentiation factor (NDF) (Wen et al. 1992), acetylcholine receptor-inducing activity (ARIA; Falls et al. 1993), or glial growth factor (Marchionni et al. 1993).

A common feature of all the mammalian members of the EGF-like growth factor family is that they are initially synthesized as larger precursor forms anchored to cell surfaces via a hydrophobic transmembrane domain. These precursor proteins are biologically active in a juxtacrine fashion (Massagué and Pandiella 1993) and need to be processed by specific enzymes to release soluble paracrine factors. The cDNA of HB-EGF predicts a 208 amino acid precursor molecule including signal sequence (Higashiyama et al. 1991) that can be processed to create multiple forms (67–86 amino acids; 19–23 kDa) of mature secreted factor (Higashiyama et al. 1992). Mature HB-EGF contains an EGF-like domain and an N-terminal, 21 amino acid stretch of predominantly basic residues that has been shown to represent the heparin-binding domain of HB-EGF (Higashiyama et al. 1993; Thompson et al. 1994). The open reading frame also encodes an N-terminal propeptide

(43–62 amino acids), a short juxtamembrane domain (12 amino acids), a hydrophobic transmembrane domain (24 amino acids) that anchors the precursor to the cell membrane, and a cytoplasmic tail (24 amino acids) that has been suggested to play a role in regulating internalization of HB-EGF (Almond and Eidels 1994).

HB-EGF is expressed in vivo predominantly by different types of muscle, brain, and epithelial tissues (Abraham et al. 1993; Elenius and Klagsbrun, unpublished). It is also found in wound fluid, probably as a product of activated macrophages (Marikovsky et al. 1993). It has been speculated that the predominant form of HB-EGF in normal, un-wounded mature tissues is the transmembrane form, whereas some non adherent cell types constitutively secrete a soluble factor (Blotnick et al. 1994; Klagsbrun 1995). Because of its nature as a potent mitogen and chemoattractant for cultured smooth muscle cells (Higashiyama et al. 1993), HB-EGF has been implicated in diseases involving smooth muscle cell hyperplasia or hypertrophy. For example, increased HB-EGF expression has been associated with atherosclerosis (Miyagawa et al. 1995) and pulmonary hypertension (Powell et al. 1993), whereas generation of uterine leiomyomas has been suggested to coincide with enhanced processing of HB-EGF precursor (Mangrulkar et al. 1995). Recent findings further indicate an involvement of transmembrane HB-EGF in the signaling and adhesion that occurs between the uterine wall and the receptors at the surface of an implanting mouse blastocyst: For example, it was found that the expression of HB-EGF precursor is induced in the uterine epithelium exclusively at sites of blastocyst apposition (Das et al. 1994). Furthermore, transmembrane HB-EGF overexpressed in a cell line mediates adhesion of the cells to blastocysts in vitro (Raab et al. 1996). A novel property of the cell-associated HB-EGF precursor is that it, but not other EGF-like ligands, functions as the receptor for *Diphtheria* toxin (Naglich et al. 1992; Iwamoto et al. 1994).

Members of the EGF-like ligand family bind to and activate members of the EGF-receptor family. At present the EGF-receptor family consists of four members: HER1/EGFR, HER2/ErbB2/*neu*, HER3/ErbB3, and HER4/ErbB4 (Hynes and Stern 1994; Earp et al. 1995). All four receptors share some structural and functional similarities, including: two cysteine-rich domains in the extracellular domain, a single membrane-spanning domain, an intracellular tyrosine kinase domain, and a C-terminal cytoplasmic tail with several binding sites for signal transduction molecules containing SH2-domains. Ligand binding to these receptors induces receptor dimerization, autophosphorylation at tyrosine residues, and internalization of the ligand–receptor complex (Ullrich and Schlessinger 1990; Schlessinger and Ullrich 1992). Heterodimerization can probably occur between any two members of the family (Riese et al., in press, 1996) and is sometimes even preferred over homodimerization in response to ligand binding (Qian et al. 1994; Karunagaran et al. 1996).

It has been suggested that members of the EGF-like ligand family can be separated into three categories based on their direct interactions with receptors (Riese et al. 1996); (1) those that bind solely to EGFR (e.g., EGF, TGF-α), (2) those that *do not* bind to EGFR (e.g., heregulin/NDF which binds HER3 and HER4), and (3) those that can bind both EGFR and another receptor (e.g., betacellulin which can independently activate both EGFR and HER4). None of the known ligands of EGF family can bind or activate HER2 in the absence of heterodimer formation with other receptors (Carraway and Cantley 1994). A feature of HB-EGF, amphiregulin, and some splice variants of NDF/heregulin not shared by other EGF family members is their affinity for heparin. The interactions of these factors with cell surface or matrix-associated heparan sulfate proteoglycans (HSPG) could further modify their accessibility or affinity for the tyrosine kinase receptors or the nature of the signal activated.

Several experiments have implicated EGFR as a receptor for HB-EGF. HB-EGF has been shown to compete for the binding of ^{125}I-labeled EGF to A431 cells (Higashiyama et al. 1991), to cross-link to a 170-kDa receptor on the surface of A431 cells, of smooth muscle cells, and of Chinese hamster ovary (CHO) cells engineered to overexpress EGFR (Higashiyama et al. 1993, 1994; Aviezer and Yayon 1994), and to activate EGFR phosphorylation in several cell types, including A431 cells, when assessed using EGFR specific antibodies (Higashiyama et al. 1992, 1994; Aviezer and Yayon 1994; Das et al. 1994). HB-EGF can also induce proliferation of interleukin-3 (IL-3) dependent cells transfected with EGFR in the absence of IL-3 both as a paracrine and as a juxtacrine factor (Higashiyama et al. 1995). The role of heparin-like molecules in HB-EGF signaling still needs to be fully elucidated but several reports demonstrate that HSPG at the cell surfaces can bind HB-EGF (Aviezer and Yayon 1994; Mesri et al. 1994; Bennett et al.

1995; Raab et al. 1996) and that HB-EGF responses are modified by the presence of heparin-like molecules (Higashiyama et al. 1993; Marik-ovsky et al. 1993; Aviezer and Yayon 1994).

The results obtained to date do not rule out the existence or even requirement of other cell surface-associated molecules participating in HB-EGF activated signal transduction. Therefore we have analyzed several cell types for their ability to cross-link HB-EGF and for their biological responses to mature HB-EGF and to HB-EGF *Pseudomonas* exotoxin (HB-EGF-PE) chimeric toxin. We report that some cell types respond differently to the mitogenic and toxic effects of HB-EGF and EGF/TGF-α and their toxin fusion proteins, respectively, and that HB-EGF forms cross-linked complexes that appear inconsistent with EGFR binding.

3.2 Materials and Methods

3.2.1 Cell Culture and [^{3}H]Thymidine Incorporation Assays

All cell lines studied were cultured in Dulbecco's modified Eagle's medium (DMEM) containing 10% fetal calf serum (FCS) and 1% glutamine/penicillin/streptomycin supplement (GPS; Irvine Scientific; Santa Ana, CA, USA) with the exception of 32D cells expressing EGFR (EP170.7) (Pierce et al. 1988). These cells, referred to here as 32D-HER1, were cultured in RPMI-1640, 10% FCS, 1% GPS and 5% WEHI-conditioned medium (Pierce et al. 1988). Before addition of growth factor, cells were split into 96-well plates and starved for 5 days in serum-free medium (A431 and HepG2 cells) or as described previously for Balb/C 3T3, bovine aortic endothelial cells (BAEC) and bovine aortic smooth muscle cells (BASMC) (Besner et al. 1990). Mitogenic assays for 32D-HER1 cells were performed as described (Blotnick et al. 1994). Recombinant human HB-EGF (obtained from Dr. J. Abraham, Scios-Nova, Mountain View, CA) or EGF (Intergen; Purchase, NJ, USA) was added for the last 24 h of the experiments. One μCi/ml of [^{3}H]thymidine (NEN) was added 6–8 h before harvesting and the amount of [^{3}H]thymidine incorporated into DNA was estimated using a Microbeta scintillation counter (Wallac; Turku, Finland).

3.2.2 Toxicity Assays for Cell Lines

Fusion proteins of HB-EGF and TGF-α coupled to *Pseudomonas* exotoxin (PE) to produce HB-EGF-PE and TGF-α-PE chimeric toxins were prepared and used to kill cells as described previously (Mesri et al. 1994). Briefly, cells were grown to confluency in 96-well plates, toxins were added for 16–18 h and for the last 2 h of the experiment 5 μCi/ml of [^{3}H]leucine (NEN) was applied to cells in leucine-free medium. Incorporated radioactivity, reflecting the amount of total protein synthesis, was assessed using a Microbeta scintillation counter (Wallac).

3.2.3 Cross-Linking for Cell Lines

Iodination of HB-EGF was performed with Iodobeads (Pierce; Rockford, IL, USA) according to the manufacturer's recommendations and a specific activity of about 100 000 cpm/ng was achieved. For cross-linking to cell surfaces, labeled HB-EGF was used in a concentration of 5 ng/ml as described (Vaisman et al. 1990). After cross-linking with disuccinimidyl suberate (DSS), cells were lysed and samples from detergent soluble fractions were analyzed on 6% sodium dodecyl sulfate polyacrylamide gel electrophoresis (SDS-PAGE) gels. The gels were dried and cross-linked complexes were visualized by autoradiography.

3.2.4 Blastocyst Experiments

To examine the effects of growth factor *Pseudomonas* toxin fusion proteins on blastocysts, mouse blastocysts were recovered on day 4 of pregnancy (1300–1400 h) and their zona pellucidae removed using 0.5% pronase treatment. Zona-free blastocysts were then cultured in groups of 6–10 in 25 μl of Whitten's medium under silicon oil in an atmosphere of 5% CO_2/95% air at 37°C for 18 h without or with various concentrations of HB-EGF-PE or TGF-α-PE. At the end of the culture, blastocysts were incubated in [^{14}C]-leucine (200 000 cpm/drop) in 25 μl medium at 37°C for 3 h. Blastocysts were washed four times with Whitten's medium and placed on glass fiber filters (GF-C, Whatman; Maidstone, UK). The filters were rapidly washed with 10 ml of 10%

trichloroacetic acid (TCA) and 20 ml of 5% TCA under vacuum. The filters were further washed with absolute alcohol, dried at 50°C for 5 min and the radioactivity measured.

For cross-linking experiments, day 4 blastocysts were collected in batches of 70 in 50 μl of binding buffer (50 mM piperazine-diethanesulfonic acid, PIPES, 0.5% BSA, 128 mM NaCl, 5 mM KCl, and 1.2 mM MgSO$_4$, pH 7.5) and sonicated. The homogenates were incubated for 2 h at room temperature in 100 μl of binding buffer containing ^{125}I-labeled HB-EGF (100 000 cpm). Samples were then diluted with 500 μl of binding buffer and centrifuged at 110 000 g for 30 min. The pellets were dissolved in 25 μl of binding buffer without BSA and cross-linking was performed for 10 min at room temperature by adding DSS (0.75 mM). Cross-linked products were extracted with 30 μl of buffer containing 10 mM tris-(hydroxymethyl)-aminomethane (Tris), 1 mM ethylene diamine tetraacetate (EDTA), 0.15 M NaCl, 1% Triton X-100 for 15 min at 4°C and centrifuged. The supernatants were then analyzed on 7.5% SDS-PAGE gels followed by autoradiography.

3.3 Results

3.3.1 Mitogenic Activity of HB-EGF

The effects of HB-EGF on DNA synthesis were measured using [^{3}H]thymidine incorporation assays. As previously described (Higashiyama et al. 1991), HB-EGF was found to be a potent mitogen for mouse Balb/C 3T3 (3T3) fibroblasts and for BASMC with ED$_{50}$ values 0.2 ng/ml and 0.6 ng/ml, respectively (Fig. 1). HB-EGF did not stimulate DNA synthesis in BAEC even at concentrations up to 100 ng/ml (Fig. 1), while 10 ng/ml of bFGF, on the other hand, stimulated a three- to fourfold increase in [^{3}H]thymidine incorporation when analyzed with the same batch of cells (not shown). Two human cell lines, a hepatoblastoma-derived HepG2 and an epidermoid carcinoma line A431, showed an inhibitory response to high (10–100 ng/ml) HB-EGF concentrations (Fig. 1). Similar results were obtained after treatment with EGF (not shown).

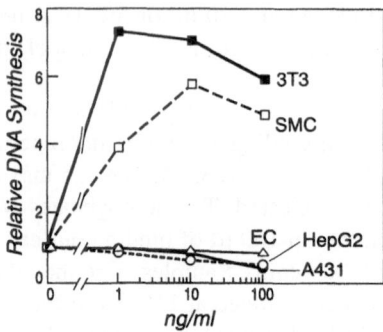

Fig. 1. Dose-dependent effects of heparin-binding EGF-like growth factor
(HB-EGF) on DNA synthesis. [^{3}H]Thymidine incorporation in response to 24
h of HB-EGF treatment was analyzed for *3T3* cells (*black squares*), bovine
aortic smooth muscle cells (*SMC, white squares*), bovine aortic endothelial
cells (*EC, white triangles*), *HepG2* cells (*white circles*), and *A431* cells (*black
circles*). Each *point* represents the mean of three parallel measurements. Total
cpm was obtained by subtracting by the values obtained for untreated cells of
the same cell line, and the data were expressed as relative DNA synthesis

3.3.2 HB-EGF-PE Toxicity for Cells

As another approach to determine biological responses that require
HB-EGF binding to cell surface molecules, the effect of HB-EGF-PE on
protein synthesis was investigated using the same five cell lines that
were used for mitogenic assays (Fig. 2). PE needs to be internalized by
specific cell surface molecules in order to enter the cytosol and arrest
protein synthesis. In HB-EGF-PE, the domain that in wild-type PE is
responsible for cell binding, is mutated, leaving the HB-EGF domain
responsible for binding to cell surfaces and mediating internalization
(Mesri et al. 1994). When analyzed 16–18 h after addition of the toxin,
protein synthesis was found to be most effectively inhibited in A431
cells with an ED_{50} of 0.02 ng/ml. The chimeric toxin was equipotent for
HepG2 and BASMC cells (ED_{50}=0.4 ng/ml) and significantly less potent for 3T3 cells (ED_{50}=10 ng/ml). BAEC were the most resistant cells
for the effect of HB-EGF-PE on protein synthesis (ED_{50}=60 ng/ml).

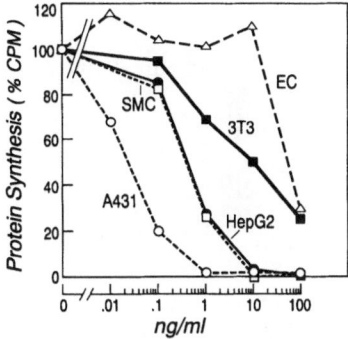

Fig. 2. Dose-dependent toxic effects of heparin-binding EGF-like growth factor *Pseudomonas* exotoxin (HB-EGF-PE) chimeric toxin on protein synthesis. Bovine aortic endothelial cells (*EC*; *white triangles*), *3T3* cells (*black squares*), HepG2 cells (*black circles*), bovine aortic smooth muscle cells (*SMC*; *white squares*) and *A431* cells (*white circles*) were analyzed for their sensitivity to treatment with indicated concentrations of toxin. The effect on protein synthesis was measured by estimating the incorporation of [^{3}H]leucine into protein. The cpm value obtained for untreated cells is expressed as 100%

3.3.3 ^{125}I-Labeled HB-EGF Cross-Linking to Cells

The same five cell lines were further subjected to cross-linking analysis with ^{125}I-labeled HB-EGF (Fig. 3). ^{125}I-labeled HB-EGF was cross-linked to form complexes of 185 kDa at the surface of all the cell lines except BAEC. This size was expected for a complex formed between a monomer of recombinant HB-EGF and a monomer of EGFR (15 kDa HB-EGF + 170 kDa EGFR). The intensity of the band was strongest for A431 cells (Fig. 3, lane 1), and was diminished in the order: HepG2 (Fig. 3, lane 4), BASMC (Fig. 3, lane 2) and 3T3 (Fig. 3, lane 5). After densitometric quantitation, the intensity of the 185-kDa band was estimated to be 100, 37, 24, 8, and 0 for A431, HepG2, BASMC, 3T3 and BAEC, respectively (relative units; A431=100).

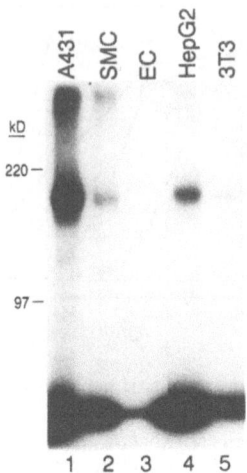

Fig. 3. Cross-linking of ^{125}I-labeled heparin-binding EGF-like growth factor (HB-EGF) to cell surfaces, whereby 5 ng/ml of ^{125}I-labeled HB-EGF was cross-linked to confluent 6-cm dishes of *A431* cells (*lane 1*), bovine aortic smooth muscle cells (*SMC; lane 2*), bovine aortic endothelial cells (*EC; lane 3*), HepG2 cells (*lane 4*), and *3T3* cells (*lane 5*). After cross-linking, cells were solubilized and samples of the same volume were loaded onto a 6% sodium dodecyl sulfate polyacrylamide gel electrophoresis gel. An autoradiogram of a dried gel is shown

3.3.4 EGFR Is Not the Optimal Receptor for HB-EGF

The results that have been obtained so far demonstrate that HB-EGF binds to the same receptor (EGFR) (Fig. 3) and has similar mitogenic effects as EGF (Fig. 1). However, when DNA synthesis was measured in an IL-3-dependent 32D cell line transfected with EGFR (Pierce et al. 1988) in the absence of IL-3, EGF was found to be reproducibly tenfold more potent than HB-EGF (ED_{50} of 0.1 ng/ml for EGF vs. ED_{50} of 1.0 ng/ml for HB-EGF) (Fig. 4a). As a control for growth factor efficacy, when samples from the same growth factor aliquots were applied to 3T3 cells, no significant differences in the potencies were observed (ED_{50} of 0.3 ng/ml for EGF vs. ED_{50} of 0.2 ng/ml for HB-EGF) (Fig. 4b).

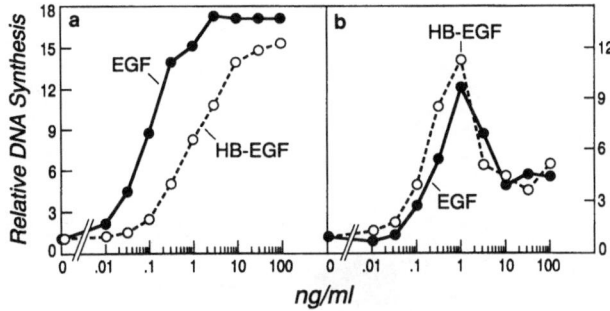

Fig. 4a,b. Comparison of the effects of heparin-binding EGF-like growth factor (*HB-EGF*) and epidermal growth factor (*EGF*) on DNA synthesis in (**a**) 32D cells transfected with EGF receptor (32D-HER1) or (**b**) in Balb/C 3T3 fibroblasts (3T3). DNA synthesis was measured as described in Fig. 1

3.3.5 ^{125}I-Labeled HB-EGF Binds to Multiple Receptors

In further support of functional differences between HB-EGF and EGF, cross-linking patterns of ^{125}I-labeled HB-EGF did not duplicate that of ^{125}I-labeled EGF in some cell lines. Although in the majority of cell lines ^{125}I-labeled HB-EGF cross-linked to cells in a similar manner to ^{125}I-labeled EGF (Fig. 3 and data not shown), cross-linking of ^{125}I-labeled HB-EGF to MDA-MB-453 human breast cancer cells resulted in two complexes of about 190 kDa and 160 kDa (Fig. 5a, lane 1). Neither of these complexes was of exactly the same size as the complex formed by cross-linking of ^{125}I-labeled HB-EGF to BASMC (Fig. 5a, lane 2) or to A431 cells (not shown). Furthermore, neither of the cross-linked complexes were formed in MDA-MB-453 cells with ^{125}I-labeled EGF (not shown). Similar results were obtained when mouse blastocysts were cross-linked with iodinated growth factors (Fig. 5b, lane 3). ^{125}I-labeled HB-EGF was cross-linked to form two complexes that were of similar size as those formed by MDA-MB-453 cells (Fig. 5a, lane 1). On the other hand, ^{125}I-labeled EGF did not cross-link mouse blastocysts (not shown).

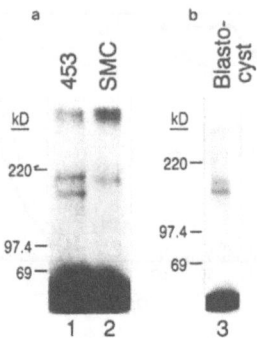

Fig. 5a,b. Cross-linking of ^{125}I-labeled heparin-binding EGF-like growth factor to MDA-MB-453 (*453*) cells (**a**, *lane 1*), bovine aortic smooth muscle cells (*SMC;* **a**, *lane 2*) or to isolated mouse blastocysts (**b**, *lane 3*). Samples were analyzed on a 6% (**a**) or on a 7.5% (**b**) sodium dodecyl sulfate polyacrylamide gel electrophoresis gel

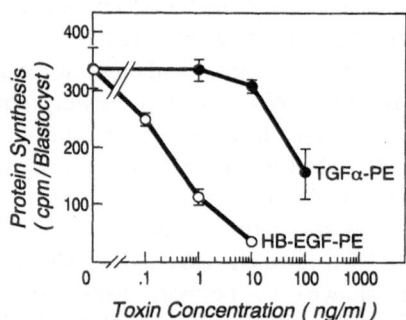

Fig. 6. Comparison of the dose-dependent effects of heparin-binding EGF-like growth factor *Pseudomonas* exotoxin (*HB-EGF-PE*) and transforming growth factor-α PE (*TGF-α-PE*) on [^{14}C]leucine incorporation into isolated mouse blastocysts. Results are expressed as cpm of incorporated [^{14}C]leucine divided by the number of blastocysts used in a sample

3.3.6 Differential HB-EGF-PE and TGF-α-PE Toxicity
for Mouse Blastocysts

To explore functional responses associated with the expression of atypical HB-EGF receptors, mouse blastocysts were analyzed for their response to HB-EGF-PE and TGF-α-PE, a chimeric toxin produced by the insertion of a TGF-α sequence to mediate cell surface binding and internalization (Mesri et al. 1994). HB-EGF-PE was shown to be significantly more potent, about two hundred-fold, in inhibiting protein synthesis in blastocysts in vitro as compared to TGF-α-PE (ED_{50} 0.5 ng/ml and 100 ng/ml for HB-EGF-PE and TGF-α-PE, respectively) (Fig. 6). These results suggest the presence of differential receptors for HB-EGF and TGF-α on mouse blastocysts.

3.4 Discussion

In order to identify receptors for the mature soluble form of HB-EGF, we analyzed the responses of five cell lines (BAEC, BASMC, 3T3, HepG2 and A431) to HB-EGF and to a chimeric toxin composed of HB-EGF and *Pseudomonas* exotoxin, HB-EGF-PE. HB-EGF responses were assessed by measuring the rate of DNA synthesis which reflects proliferation, and HB-EGF-PE responses were assessed by estimating [^{3}H]leucine incorporation which reflects the ability of the toxin to inhibit protein synthesis. In addition, the five cell lines were cross-linked with ^{125}I-labeled HB-EGF which formed complexes with EGFR. Interestingly, there was very little correlation between the mitogenic effects of HB-EGF and the toxic effects of HB-EGF-PE. In fact, these biological assays seemed to yield inverse results (Table 1). For example, HB-EGF was very mitogenic for 3T3 cells but HB-EGF-PE was a relatively poor toxin for these cells. On the other hand, there was an excellent correlation between toxicity and the number of cell surface receptors found on a given cell type as determined by ^{125}I-labeled HB-EGF cross-linking (Table 1). For example, A431 cells which expressed the most cross-linkable cell surface receptors were the most sensitive to HB-EGF-PE-induced toxicity (ED_{50} 0.02 ng/ml) but their growth was actually inhibited by HB-EGF. These results suggest that cross-linking and toxin assays measure receptor binding; on the other

Table 1. Comparison of EGFR cross-linking levels, HB-EGF-PE toxicity and HB-EGF mitogenicity

Cell line	Relative EGFR cross-linking (% of A431)	HB-EGF-PE ED_{50} (ng/ml)	HB-EGF ED_{50} (ng/ml)
EC	0	60	–
3T3	8	10	0.2
SMC	24	0.4	0.6
HepG2	32	0.4	10–100 (Inh.)
A431	100	0.02	10–100 (Inh.)

Cross-linking intensity was determined by densitometric quantitation of the 125I-labeled heparin-binding EGF-like growth factor (HB-EGF) cross-linking results shown in Fig. 3 (the signal for A431 cells is expressed as 100%). The ED_{50} for HB-EGF-*Pseudomonas* exotoxin (HB-EGF-PE) and HB-EGF represents the concentration (ng/ml) at which half of the maximal response was obtained when analyzed by [³H]leucine or [³H]thymidine incorporation, respectively.

–, no effect; Inh., inhibitory effect; EC, bovine aortic endothelial cells; SMC, bovine aortic smooth muscle cells.

hand, a more complex and cell type-specific signal transduction is needed to regulate cellular proliferation. These results also emphasize the inadequacy of mitogenic assays as a sole measurement for the expression of functional growth factor receptors.

Although a large number of HB-EGF-responsive cell lines were found to express a receptor with the predicted size of EGFR as their only 125I-labeled HB-EGF-binding cell surface molecule, there are several indications that EGFR is not necessarily the optimal receptor for HB-EGF and that HB-EGF also interacts with other receptors. For example, HB-EGF was found to be a far less potent mitogen (about tenfold) than EGF for 32D cells transfected with EGFR although these two factors showed quantitatively similar effects in 3T3 cells. Since 32D cells do not appear to express HSPG on their surfaces and the wild-type cells do not respond to either EGF or HB-EGF, the mitogenic response of 32D-HER1 cells to EGF-family ligands is considered to represent pure activation of EGFR without other contributing factors. On the other hand, other cell types such as 3T3 fibroblasts which express HSPG and possibly other receptor molecules might have an enhanced HB-EGF response in comparison to 32D-HER1 cells. Heparin-like molecules have indeed been demonstrated to enhance the capability of HB-EGF to induce keratinocyte proliferation (Marikovsky et al. 1993) or to bind and phosphorylate EGFR in transfected CHO cells (Aviezer and Yayon 1994). Furthermore, we have recently found a binding site for an epitope tagged HB-EGF construct at the apical site of proximal kidney tubules that can be competed with an excess of wild-type HB-EGF but not with EGF (Elenius and Klagsbrun, unpublished). As EGFR in these cells is polarized to basal surfaces, this novel binding site possibly represents a HSPG or a high-affinity receptor other than EGFR.

We have suggestive evidence that HB-EGF might recognize receptors different than those recognized by EGF or TGF-α. For example, HB-EGF-PE is 200-fold more toxic for mouse blastocysts than is TGF-α-PE (ED$_{50}$ of 0.5 ng/ml vs. 100 ng/ml, respectively). Since it appears that toxicity is a measure of binding intensity, these results suggest that mouse blastocysts express receptors that are recognized by HB-EGF but not readily by TGF-α. Although some of this differential might be accounted for by HSPG, proteoglycans alone cannot account for the whole differential (Dey et al., unpublished). Other experiments suggest that HB-EGF forms atypical complexes. Cross-linking of HB-EGF to MDA-MB-453 cells and isolated mouse blastocysts detects, in both cases, two complexes (180–190 kDa and 150–160 kDa) that do not co-migrate with the 185-kDa complex formed with BASMC EGFR. These atypically sized complexes do not appear to contain HSPG since the experimental conditions of cross-linking would not preserve HS–protein interactions and the bands formed on the SDS-PAGE gel are too sharp. One possibility is that HB-EGF is binding to HER4 on these cells. MDA-MB-453 cells have undetectable levels of EGFR but over-express HER4 (Plowman et al. 1993) and our preliminary studies with a HER4-transfected cell line suggest that HB-EGF can both bind and phosphorylate HER4 in an EGFR-independent manner (Elenius and Klagsbrun, unpublished). No data about the expression pattern of HER4 in blastocyst trophoectodermal cells have been reported to date but homozygous HER4 knockout mice did not seem to have any disadvantage at this stage of development (Gassmann et al. 1995). This could be explained by molecular redundancy since HER4 is not the only HB-EGF binding molecule. EGFR is known to be expressed within the implanting blastocyst (Paria et al. 1993) but could be polarized to the basal surface (Dardik et al. 1992) and thus possibly incapable of interacting with HB-EGF expressed in the uterine epithelium. In any case, the molecular identities of the two complexes formed by cross-linking of ^{125}I-labeled HB-EGF to blastocysts have not yet been demonstrated and need to be characterized in future experiments.

Taken together, HB-EGF seems to be able to bind to at least three different types of cell surface molecules: EGFR, HER4, and HSPG. This would justify the classification of HB-EGF in the group of EGF-like ligands, represented at the moment by betacellulin (Riese et al. 1996), that can bind or activate independently both EGFR and HER4. However, HB-EGF would thus be the only characterized ligand that can activate these two different receptor systems in a HSPG-regulated manner, giving rise to several possible modifications in the signal transduction pathways and biological responses, depending on the molecular combinations expressed at the target cell.

Acknowledgements. This work was supported by NIH grants GM 47397 (M. K.), HD 29968 and HD 12304 (S. K. D.) and by the Finnish Cultural Foundation (K. E.).

References

Abraham JA, Damm D, Bajardi A, Miller J, Klagsbrun M, Ezekowitz RA (1993) Heparin-binding EGF-like growth factor: characterization of rat and mouse cDNA clones, protein domain conservation across species, and transcript expression in tissues. Biochem Biophys Res Commun 190:125–133

Almond BD, Eidels L (1994) The cytoplasmic domain of the diphtheria toxin receptor (HB-EGF precursor) is not required for receptor-mediated endocytosis. J Biol Chem 269:26635–26641

Aviezer D, Yayon A (1994) Heparin-dependent binding and autophosphorylation of epidermal growth factor (EGF) receptor by heparin-binding EGF-like growth factor but not by EGF. Proc Natl Acad Sci USA 91:12173–12177

Bennett KL, Jackson DG, Simon JC, Tanczos E, Peach R, Modrell B, Stamenkovic I, Plowman G, Aruffo A (1995) CD44 isoforms containing exon V3 are responsible for the presentation of heparin-binding growth factor. J Cell Biol 128:687–698

Besner G, Higashiyama S, Klagsbrun M (1990) Isolation and characterization of a macrophage-derived heparin-binding growth factor. Cell Regul 1:811–819

Blotnick S, Peoples GE, Freeman MR, Eberlein TJ, Klagsbrun M (1994) T lymphocytes synthesize and export heparin-binding epidermal growth factor-like growth factor and basic fibroblast growth factor, mitogens for vascular cells and fibroblasts: differential production and release by CD4+ and CD8+ T cells. Proc Natl Acad SCI USA 91:2890–2894

Carraway KL, Cantley LC (1994) A neu acquaintance for erbB3 and erbB4: a role for receptor heterodimerization in growth signaling. Cell 78:5–8

Cohen S, Carpenter G, King L Jr (1980) Epidermal growth factor-receptor-protein kinase interactions. Co-purification of receptor and epidermal growth factor-enhanced phosphorylation activity. J Biol Chem 255:4834–4842

Dardik A, Smith RM, Schultz RM (1992) Colocalization of transforming growth factor-α and a functional epidermal growth factor receptor (EGFR) to the inner cell mass and preferential localization of the EGFR on the basolateral surface of the trophectoderm in the mouse blastocyst. Dev Biol 154:393–409

Das SK, Wang XN, Paria BC, Damm D, Abraham JA, Klagsbrun M, Andrews GK, Dey SK (1994) Heparin-binding EGF-like growth factor gene is induced in the mouse uterus temporally by the blastocyst solely at the site of its apposition: a possible ligand for interaction with blastocyst EGF-receptor in implantation. Development 120:1071–1083

Derynck R, Roberts AB, Winkler ME, Chen EY, Goeddel DV (1984) Human transforming growth factor-alpha: precursor structure and expression in E. coli. Cell 38:287–297

Earp HS, Dawson TL, Li X, Yu H (1995) Heterodimerization and functional interaction between EGF receptor family members: a new signaling paradigm with implications for breast cancer research. Breast Cancer Res Treat 35:115–132

Falls DL, Rosen KM, Corfas G, Lane WS, Fischbach GD (1993) ARIA, a protein that stimulates acetylcholine receptor synthesis, is a member of the neu ligand family. Cell 72:801–815

Gassmann M, Casagranda F, Orioli D, Simon H, Lai C, Klein R, Lemke G (1995) Aberrant neural and cardiac development in mice lacking the ErbB4 neuregulin receptor. Nature 378:390–394

Higashiyama S, Abraham JA, Miller J, Fiddes JC, Klagsbrun M (1991) A heparin-binding growth factor secreted by macrophage-like cells that is related to EGF. Science 251:936–939

Higashiyama S, Lau K, Besner GE, Abraham JA, Klagsbrun M (1992) Structure of heparin-binding EGF-like growth factor. Multiple forms, primary structure, and glycosylation of the mature protein. J Biol Chem 267:6205–6212

Higashiyama S, Abraham JA, Klagsbrun M (1993) Heparin-binding EGF-like growth factor stimulation of smooth muscle cell migration: dependence on interactions with cell surface heparan sulfate. J Cell Biol 122:933–940

Higashiyama S, Abraham JA, Klagsbrun M (1994) Heparin-binding EGF-like growth factor synthesis by smooth muscle cells. Horm Res 42:9–13

Higashiyama S, Iwamoto R, Goishi K, Raab G, Taniguchi N, Klagsbrun M, Mekada E (1995) The membrane protein CD9/DRAP 27 potentiates the juxtacrine growth factor activity of the membrane-anchored heparin-binding EGF-like growth factor. J Cell Biol 128:929–938

Holmes WE, Sliwkowski MX, Akita RW, Henzel WJ, Lee J, Park JW, Yansura D, Abadi N, Raab H, Lewis GD, Shepard HM, Kuang W-J, Wood WI, Goeddel DV, Vandlen RL (1992) Identification of heregulin, a specific activator of p185erbB2. Science 256:1205–1210

Hynes NE, Stern DF (1994) The biology of erbB-2/neu/HER-2 and its role in cancer. Biochim Biophys Acta 1198:165–184

Iwamoto R, Higashiyama S, Mitamura T, Taniguchi N, Klagsbrun M, Mekada E (1994) Heparin-binding EGF-like growth factor, which acts as the diphtheria toxin receptor, forms a complex with membrane protein DRAP27/CD9, which up-regulates functional receptors and diphtheria toxin sensitivity. EMBO J 13:2322–2330

Karunagaran D, Tzahar E, Beerli RR, Chen X, Graus-Porta D, Ratzkin BJ, Seger R, Hynes NE, Yarden Y (1996) ErbB-2 is a common auxiliary subunit of NDF and EGF receptors: implications for breast cancer. EMBO J 15:254–264

Kimura H, Fischer WH, Schubert D (1990) Structure, expression and function of a schwannoma-derived growth factor. Nature 348:257–260

Klagsbrun M (1995) The structural and biological properties of the transmembrane and mature forms of heparin-binding EGF-like growth factor. In: Orosz CG, Dedmark DD, Ferguson RM (eds) Transplant vascular sclerosis. Springer, New York, pp 141–150

Mangrulkar RS, Ono M, Ishikawa M, Takashima S, Klagsbrun M, Nowak RA (1995) Isolation and characterization of heparin-binding growth factors in human leiomyomas and normal myometrium. Biol Reprod 53:636–646

Marchionni MA, Goodearl ADJ, Chen MS, Bermingham-McDonogh O, Kirk C, Hendricks M, Danehy F, Misumi D, Sudhalter J, Kobayashi K, Wroblewski D, Lynch C, Baldassare M, Hiles I, Davis JB, Hsuan JJ, Totty NF, Otsu M, McBurney RN, Waterfield MD, Stroobant P, Gwynne D (1993) Glial growth factors are alternatively spliced erbB2 ligands expresses in the nervous system. Nature 362:312–318

Marikovsky M, Breuing K, Liu PY, Eriksson E, Higashiyama S, Farber P, Abraham J, Klagsbrun M (1993) Appearance of heparin-binding EGF-like growth factor in wound fluid as a response to injury. Proc Natl Acad Sci USA 90:3889–3893

Massagué J, Pandiella A (1993) Membrane-anchored growth factors. Annu Rev Biochem 62:515–541

Mesri EA, Ono M, Kreitman RJ, Klagsbrun M, Pastan I (1994) The heparin-binding domain of heparin-binding EGF-like growth factor can target Pseudomonas exotoxin to kill cells exclusively through heparan sulfate proteoglycans. J Cell Sci 107:2599–2608

Miyagawa J, Higashiyama S, Kawata S, Inui Y, Tamura S, Yamamoto K, Nishida M, Nakamura T, Yamashita S, Matsuzawa Y, Taniguchi N (1995) Localization of heparin-binding EGF-like growth factor in the smooth muscle cells and macrophages of human atherosclerotic plaques. J Clin Invest 95:404–411

Naglich JG, Metherall JE, Russell DW, Eidels L (1992) Expression cloning of a diphtheria toxin receptor: identity with a heparin-binding EGF-like growth factor precursor. Cell 69:1051–1061

Paria BC, Das SK, Andrews GK, Dey SK (1993) Expression of the epidermal growth factor receptor gene is regulated in mouse blastocysts during delayed implantation. Proc Natl Acad Sci USA 90:55–59

Pierce JH, Ruggiero M, Fleming TP, Di Fiore PP, Greenberger JS, Varticovski L, Schlessinger J, Rovera G, Aaronson SA (1988) Signal transduction through the EGF receptor transfected in IL-3-dependent hematopoietic cells. Science 239:628–631

Plowman GD, Culouscou DIM, Whitney GS, Green JM, Carlton GW, Foy L, Neubauer MG, Shoyab M (1993) Ligand-specific activation of HER4/p180erbB4, a fourth member of the epidermal growth factor receptor family. Proc Natl Acad Sci USA 90:1746–1750

Powell PP, Klagsbrun M, Abraham JA, Jones RC (1993) Eosinophils expressing heparin-binding EGF-like growth factor mRNA localize around lung microvessels in pulmonary hypertension. Am J Pathol 143:784–793

Qian X, LeVea CM, Freeman JK, Dougall WC, Greene MI (1994) Heterodimerization of epidermal growth factor receptor and wild type or kinase-deficient neu: a mechanism of interreceptor kinase activation and transphosphorylation. Proc Natl Acad Sci USA 91:1500–1504

Raab G, Kover K, Paria BC, Dey SK, Ezzell RM, Klagsbrun M (1996) Mouse preimplantation blastocysts adhere to cells expressing the transmembrane form of heparin-binding EGF-like growth factor. Development 122:637–645

Riese DJ, Bermingham Y, van Raaij TM, Buckley S, Plowman GD, Stern DF (1996) Betacellulin activates the epidermal growth factor receptor and erbB-4, and induces cellular response patterns distinct from those stimulated by epidermal growth factor or neuregulin-β. Oncogene 12:345–353

Savage CR Jr, Inagami T, Cohen S (1972) The primary structure of epidermal growth factor. J Biol Chem 247:7612–7621

Schlessinger J, Ullrich A (1992) Growth factor signaling by receptor tyrosine kinases. Neuron 9:383–391

Shing Y, Christofori G, Hanahan D, Ono Y, Sasada R, Igarashi K, Folkman J (1993) Betacellulin: a mitogen from pancreatic beta cell tumors. Science 259:1604–1607

Shoyab M, Plowman GD, McDonald VL, Bradley JG, Todaro GJ (1989) Structure and function of human amphiregulin: a member of the epidermal growth factor family. Science 243:1074–1076

Thompson SA, Higashiyama S, Wood K, Pollitt NS, Damm D, McEnroe G, Garrick B, Ashton N, Lau K, Hancock N, Klagsbrun M, Abraham JA (1994) Characterization of sequences within heparin-binding EGF-like growth factor that mediate interaction with heparin. J Biol Chem 269:2541–2549

Toyoda H, Komurasaki T, Uchida D, Takayama Y, Isobe T, Okuyama T, Hanada K (1995) Epiregulin. A novel epidermal growth factor with mitogenic activity for rat primary hepatocytes. J Biol Chem 270:7495–7500

Ullrich A, Schlessinger J (1990) Signal transduction by receptors with tyrosine kinase activity. Cell 61:203–212

Vaisman N, Gosporadowicz D, Neufeld G (1990) Characterization of the receptors for vascular endothelial growth factor. J Biol Chem 265:19461–19466

Wen D, Peles E, Cupples R, Suggs SV, Bacus SS, Luo Y, Trail G, Hu S, Silbiger SM, Levy RB, Koski RA, Lu HS, Yarden Y (1992) Neu differentiation factor: a transmembrane glycoprotein containing an EGF domain and an immunoglobulin homology unit. Cell 69:559–572

4 Epidermal Growth Factor Receptor Expression in Head and Neck Tumorigenesis and Saturation of EGFR with Monoclonal Antibody RG83852

D.M. Shin, R. Perez-Soler, W.N. Hittelman, and W.K. Hong

4.1 Introduction

The survival rates of patients with head and neck squamous cell carcinoma have improved only marginally over the past two decades despite some improvements in diagnosis and therapeutic modalities. Chemoprevention as a means of reducing the incidence and mortality of this cancer has been extensively explored (Meyskens 1990; Lippman et al. 1994; Hong et al. 1990). Chemoprevention trials, however, have been hampered by feasibility problems associated with requiring large sample sizes and relying on cancer incidence as the study end point for determining preventive efficacy. These problems can be overcome by incorporating biomarker analyses that, by identifyng the risk of tumor

development, can be used as intermediate end points in these chemoprevention trials (Lippman et al. 1990; Shin et al. 1994b). The basis for the
development of biomarkers for upper aerodigestive tract chemoprevention trials is the understanding that the whole epithelial lining of the tract
shares a common carcinogenic exposure, resulting in an increased cancer risk throughout the exposed epithelum. This entire epithelium was
first described as "condemned mucosa" associated with "field cancerization" by Slaughter et al. in 1953 on the basis of the findings of diffuse
histologic abnormalities and multifocal squamous cell carcinomas of
the head and neck. This hypothesis is further supported clinically by the
frequent association of tumors with premalignant lesions in the same
field [e.g., oral leukoplakia (Silverman et al. 1984) or bronchial metaplasia and/or dysplasia (Auerbach et al. 1961)] and by the synchronous
or metachronous development of multiple primary tumors (Lippman
and Hong 1989).

Another concept of carcinogenesis of head and neck that underlies
biomarker utility is that of the multistep tumorigenesis process (Farber
1984). The driving force behind this process is thought to be the accumulation of genetic damage caused by continuous exposure to carcinogens (e.g., tobacco and alcohol). This damage may eventually lead to
specific genetic alterations which cause phenotypic changes in the tissues which are associated with the tumorigenesis process, such as dysregulation of cell proliferation, alterations of growth factors and their
receptors, i.e., epidermal growth factor (EGF) and its receptor (EGFR),
and alterations in other proto-oncogenes and tumor suppressor genes
(Shin et al. 1994b). EGFR is a glycoprotein (M_r 170 000) with an
intrinsic tyrosine-specific protein kinase activity encoded by the ErbB1
oncogene (Yamamoto et al. 1983). EGFR is thought to play a role in the
signal transduction pathway for transforming growth factor-α (TGF-α)
(Derynek 1988). Activation of the EGFR kinase results in both autophosphorylation and phosphorylation of tyrosine residues of several
proteins in vitro (Cohen et al. 1980; Ushiro and Cohen 1980; Cohen et
al. 1985) that are thought to play a role in cell division and differentiation.

Evidence for the role of EGFR in tumorigenesis is provided by
several observations. First, the overexpression of EGFR or one of its
ligands (EGF or TGF-α) in transfected cells is associated with malignant transformation (Velu et al. 1987). Second, high copy number of the

EGFR gene has been found in primary brain tumors of glial origin (Libermann et al. 1985) and in several other tumor types, including bladder transitional cell carcinomas (Gusterson et al. 1984), breast carcinomas (Filmus et al. 1985; Hendler and Ozanne 1984), squamous cell carcinomas of the lungs (Cerny et al. 1986; Eisbruch et al. 1987) and head and neck, and their cell lines (Todd et al. 1989; Ozanne et al. 1986; Maxwell et al. 1989; Weichselbaum et al. 1989; Santini et al. 1991).

Few data are available regarding the frequency and timing of EGFR dysregulation in the normal and premalignant epithelium adjacent to tumors during the process of tumor initiation. This paper focuses on this dysregulation of EGFR expression during the tumorigenesis process (i.e., in the hamster buccal pouch tumor model, in premalignant lesions of the head and neck, and in oral leukoplakia lesions derived from chemoprevention clinical trials). We also describe biomarker studies associated with early clinical studies exploring the use of the monoclonal anti-EGFR antibody RG 83852 for the treatment of human malignancies.

The working hypothesis behind these studies is that those individuals with premalignant lesions that exhibit a high degree of EGFR alterations (and/or other genetic or phenotypic markers) are at increased risk for progression to malignancy in the carcinogen-exposed field. Furthermore, if these markers were modulable by chemopreventive agents (i.e., retinoids), they could serve as intermediate markers of response or progression in chemoprevention trials. Moreover, it might be possible that a dysregulated gene product such as EGFR could serve as a target for chemopreventive intervention.

4.2 EGFR in the Hamster Buccal Pouch Model

The Syrian golden hamster buccal pouch model is useful for the study of oral carcinogenesis, since it closely mimics events involved in the development of precancerous lesions and squamous cell carcinomas in human head and neck tissues. This model was initially developed by Salley (1954, 1957), who experimentally produced squamous cell carcinoma in the buccal pouch, and the model was extended and standardized by Morris (1961) to more uniformly reproduce the induced lesions. Shklar and others have extensively explored and characterized the model and have used it to demonstrate the experimental efficacy of many potential chemopreventive agents (Silverman and Shklar 1963; Shklar 1965, 1982; Tsiklakis et al. 1987; Suda et al. 1986; Schwartz and Shklar 1988; Trickler and Shklar 1987; Schwartz et al. 1988).

For our own studies, a potent carcinogen, 7, 12-dimethylbenz(a)anthracene (DMBA), in a 0.5% solution in heavy mineral oil was applied to the right buccal pouch of the hamster oral mucosa three times per week up to 16 weeks. The control group of animals had mineral oil only applied in their buccal pouch for the same period of time. The animals treated with DMBA were killed after 0, 4, 8, and 16 weeks of treatment to assess the tumors' histologic characteristics and EGFR status as described elsewhere (Tsiklakis et al. 1987). All experimental conditions have been described elsewhere in detail (Shin et al. 1994a). For EGFR immunohistochemical staining, buccal pouch mucosal tissues were fixed in a 10% formalin solution and embedded in paraffin. Four micrometer tissue sections were subjected to immunohistochemical staining using monoclonal anti-EGFR antibody (mouse IgG1 from C57BL/6 mice bearing the 29.1 hybridoma; ICN Immunobiologicals, Lisle, IL, USA). Immunolocalization was performed with Vector laboratories' avidin-biotin complex (ABC) kit (Burlingame, CA, USA) per manufacturer's instructions.

The histologic examination revealed that, at the end of 4 weeks, five of 20 (25%) DMBA-treated animals showed hyperplasia with hyperkeratosis, while the other 15 animals still had normal mucosa. At the end of 8 weeks, seven of 20 animals had developed papillomas with dysplastic changes, and the other 13 had hyperplastic changes. Fifteen of 17 (88%) animals treated with DMBA had developed squamous cell carcinomas, and the remaining two exhibited dysplasia with papillomatous lesions.

None of the ten control animals showed EGFR expression in the mucosal epithelia. The epithelium treated with DMBA for 4 weeks showed focal expression of EGFR in basal and superficial layers in both normal epithelia and hyperplastic lesions, although EGFR expression was higher in hyperplastic lesions than in histologically normal epithelia. After 8 weeks of DMBA, EGFR expression was elevated markedly in the DMBA-induced dysplastic lesions of seven animals. Squamous cell carcinomas that developed after 16 weeks of DMBA treatment showed a very high level of EGFR expression in a heterogenous manner; one area showed high EGFR expression and another area in the same tumor section no expression. We also performed nonradioactive in situ hybridization for expression of EGFR mRNA on the same histologic sections. EGFR mRNA expression was well correlated with EGFR protein expression determined by immunohistochemistry.

Our results were in agreement with those of other investigators (Wong and Biswas 1986; Wong 1987), which indicated that squamous cell carcinomas induced by 16 weeks of DMBA treatment expressed a high level of EGFR protein and amplification of the gene in tumors and an established cell line (HCPC-1). More interesting was our finding that premalignant lesions (i.e., hyperplasia and dysplasia) expressed EGFR at high levels in a focal manner. These results support the concept of carcinogenesis as a multistep process. In particular, we observed heterogenous expression of EGFR (one area showed positive expression of the gene and another did not express it at all) in both premalignant lesions and squamous cell carcinomas. One may speculate that certain tumor clones can be initiated from the premalignant lesions and eventually progress to malignant tumors. Further study is needed to prove this hypothesis.

4.3 EGFR Expression in a Multistep Model of Head and Neck Carcinogenesis

To examine whether EGFR expression is dysregulated in premalignant lesions during human head and neck tumorigenesis and when these changes occur, we obtained 36 formalin-fixed, paraffin- embedded specimens of squamous cell carcinomas. All tumor specimens were selected because they also contained normal epithelium adjacent to tumors, hyperplasia, or dysplasia in the same tissue sections. Biopsy specimens of oral epithelium obtained from four normal individuals (i.e., cancer-free, nonsmoking volunteers) were used as normal controls. Four-micrometer tissue sections were mounted on aminoalkylsilane-coated slides along with paraffin-embedded 886 cells which expressed EGFR and served as internal controls for measurements of EGFR expression by image analysis. Anti-EGFR monoclonal antibody (clone E30) was obtained from BioGenex, Inc. (San Ramon, CA, USA). Immunohistochemical staining was performed with a modification of the avidin–biotin immunoperoxidase method described elsewhere (Gown and Vogel 1984). Image analysis of EGFR expression to quantitate the amount of the protein was described elsewhere (Shin et al. 1994c). The amount of EGFR expression was normalized to the internal control, 886 cells.

Of the 36 tumor samples analyzed, 28 exhibited histologically normal epithelium adjacent to tumors, 15 hyperplasia, and 24 dysplasia. The four normal (control) oral mucosa specimens all showed minimal but detectable levels of membrane-associated EGFR. In contrast, histologically normal epithelia adjacent to tumors revealed somewhat increased levels of EGFR and the EGFR protein expanded into parabasal layers. Image analysis showed that normal epithelia adjacent to tumors expressed EGFR at levels twice those of the normal controls ($p=0.021$). These results indicate that, despite histologic similarity to control epithelium, normal epithelium in the field of head and neck tumors has undergone some genetic alteration.

When we analyzed EGFR expression in adjacent normal epithelia, hyperplasia, and dysplasia, we found that EGFR levels remained elevated as the tissue progressed. However, EGFR levels increased dramatically from dysplasia to squamous cell carcinomas. The relative staining intensity (RSI) of EGFR expression reflected exactly this gross observation, where the mean values of RSI were 0.38 in normal controls, 0.78 in normal epithelium adjacent to tumors ($p=0.021$), 0.64 in hyperplasia, and 0.71 in dysplasia. The mean RSI increased significantly from dysplasia to squamous cell carcinoma (0.71 to 1.16, $p=0.01$). This apparent increase in mean EGFR expression was due not only to an increase in the number of positive (EGFR-expressing) cells but also to an increase in the number of cases with highly elevated EGFR expression in squamous cell carcinoma; five of 24 (21%) of the dysplasia specimens had on RSI of greater than 1.00, whereas 23 of 36 (64%) of the squamous cell carcinomas had an RSI of greater than 1.00.

4.4 EGFR Expression in Oral Premalignant Lesions

Since EGFR expression was increased in premalignant lesions in the multistep model of head and neck carcinogenesis, EGFR might be useful as a biomarker of risk and response to chemopreventive therapy.

The tissues whose analyses are described here were obtained from the baseline samples of a prospective chemoprevention trial. We obtained 62 oral leukoplakia samples (i.e., leukoplakia or erythroplakia) from 52 patients who were treated with either 13-*cis* retinoic acid or retinyl palmitate plus beta-carotene for 3 years. All samples were analyzed for EGFR and proliferating cell nuclear antigen (PCNA) expression. PCNA is a 36-kDa nuclear protein whose expression is associated with the late G_1 and S phases of the cell cycle and which plays a critical role in the initiation of cell proliferation (Jaskulski et al. 1988). It may be hypothesized that only those cells with high proliferative activity could be associated with tumor progression during tumorigenesis. Histologic analysis showed that 45 samples (72%) displayed hyperplasia, 12 (19%), mild dysplasia, four (7%), moderate dysplasia, and one, severe dysplasia (2%). To detect EGFR expression, we performed image analysis for all premalignant lesions after immunohistochemical staining was done as described earlier (Shin et al. 1994c). PCNA expression was quantitated by using a labeling index (LI) after immunohistochemical staining was performed, as described previously (Shin et al. 1993). LI represents the fraction of positive PCNA-expressing cells among the total counted cells.

The mean values of RSI of EGFR expression were 0.38 (± S.D., 0.07) in the four control specimens and increased to 0.67 (± S.D., 0.39) in 42 hyperplasias (*p* 0.05), 0.86 (± S.D., 0.45) in 11 mild dysplasias, 0.69 (± S.D., 0.09) in four moderate dysplasias, and 0.80 in one severe dysplasia. These results confirmed our previous findings that EGFR expression in oral premalignant lesions increased twofold from normal control epithelia to hyperplasia and stayed high in mild, moderate, and severe dysplasia. Since all tissue samples were from premalignant lesions, no values were obtained for tumors.

When PCNA expression was analyzed in different histologic tissue types, mean values of LI of PCNA expression were 0.04 (± S.D., 0.01) in six normal controls, 0.14 (± S.D., 0.09) in 35 hyperplasias, 0.35 (± S.D., 0.18) in eight mild dysplasias, 0.35 (± S.D. 0.33) in two moderate dysplasias, and 0.33 in one severe dysplasia. These data indicate that there is a significant increase of PCNA expression from normal controls to hyperplasia (*p*=0.005) and a further increase from hyperplasia to mild dysplasia (*p*=0.003).

We have already demonstrated that there is biological difference between normal control epithelia from nonrisk individuals (i.e., noncancerous nonsmokers) and histologically "normal" epithelia from high-risk individuals; both PCNA and EGFR expression were increased in high-risk individuals. A question that arises is whether there is any difference in EGFR or PCNA expression in hyperplasia alone compared to that in hyperplasia adjacent to dysplasia. There is no such difference in EGFR expression (p=0.403), although we did find a significant increase in PCNA expression from hyperplasia alone to hyperplasia adjacent to dysplasia (p=0.005). These results clearly indicate that a proliferation marker (i.e., PCNA) depicts a biological difference even in the same histologic feature.

To determine whether EGFR or PCNA expression level was correlated with smoking status or alcohol consumption, we used the Wilcoxon rank-sums test tocompare EGFR or PCNA status with smoking or alcohol status. There were no significant differences in EGFR or PCNA status by smoking or alcohol status. When EGFR was compared to PCNA for each case, it did not seem to be any correlation between these two markers.

4.5 EGFR Saturation Study
with Monoclonal Antibody RG83852

Anti-EGFR monoclonal antibodies have been effective tools for examining the biochemical mechanism of EGFR action (Gill et al. 1984) and imaging EGFR-expressing tumors in humans (Divigi et al. 1991). Anti-EGFR monoclonal antibodies have been shown to inhibit growth of EGFR-expressing tumors in nude mice (Masui et al. 1984). Furthermore, these antibodies may be important modulators of EGFR expression (Christen et al. 1990) and may also increase the susceptibility to chemotherapy or radiotherapy in vitro (Kwok and Sutherland 1989, 1991).

RG83852 is an intact murine monoclonal immunoglobulin G-2a (IgG2a) antibody that recognizes an extracellular domain on EGFR and reacts with most epithelial surfaces. In particular, it reacts with 80% of human non-small-cell lung cancers and head and neck cancers (Lax et al. 1989). RG83852 has been shown to inhibit growth of KB squamous cell carcinoma xenografts in nude mice and to enhance the in vivo antitumor activity of chemotherapeutic agents, including cisplatin, in nude mice bearing KB tumors (Aboud-Pirak et al. 1988, 1989).

We conducted a phase I clinical study to define the modulation of tyrosine kinase activity, tumor EGFR saturation, and toxicity to humans associated with different doses of monoclonal antibody RF83852. A part of the results was reported previously (Perez-Soler et al. 1994).

In this report, we will describe the tissue saturation of EGFR by the monoclonal antibody RG83852 as determined by immunohistochemistry and image analysis. To be eligible for this phase I study, the patients must have had a histologic diagnosis of non-small-cell lung cancer or head and neck cancer, not have responded to standard therapy, have had a good performance status (Zubrod scale, < 2), have had disease that could be biopsied, have had adequate major organ function, and have signed a written informed consent. EGFR expression was not an eligibility criterion, since RG83852 has been shown to recognize approximately 80% of non-small-cell lung and head and neck cancers. RG83852, manufactured by Rhone-Poulenc/Rorer (Collegeville, PA, USA) and supplied by the National Cancer Institute (Bethesda, MD, USA), was administered by continuous intravenous infusion for 5 days. The starting total dose was 50 mg/m^2, and the total dose gradually increased to 100, 200, 400, and 600 mg/m^2 in each cohort of patients. Three patients were entered at each dose level and were observed for a minimum of 2 weeks before dose escalation in the next cohort.

After 5 days of infusion of RG83852, tumor tissues were obtained on day 6 (24 h after completion of infusion) from ten patients (Table 1). Pretherapy fresh tumor samples were obtained from five patients (Nos. 10, 12, 13, 14, 15), and another posttreatment tumor sample was obtained from one patient on day 9 (No. 14). Paraffin-embedded tumor samples at the time of initial diagnosis (Nos. 2 and 9) were used as pretherapy specimens for immunohistochemical analysis. Two posttherapy day 6 specimens (Nos. 5 and 8) were all necrotic tissue and could not be used for tumor EGFR saturation analysis. The nature of necrosis was not clear, whether it was related to the therapy or to the aspiration artifact, since pretreatment biopsy was not performed in these cases. In one case (No. 12), the normal skin was contained in the surgical specimen, and another case (No. 13) had normal skin on posttherapy day 6.

Table 1. Characteristics of tumor tissues

Patient No.	Histologic type	Timing of Biopsy			Dose of RG83852 (mg/m^2)	Remarks
		Treatment	Day 6	Other		
1	Adenocarcinoma of lung	ND	FNAB of lung	ND	50	Necrotic tissue
2	Squamous cell carcinoma of lung	ND	ExB of subcutaneous metastasis	ND	50	Viable tissue
3	Adenocarcinoma of the lung	ND	ExB of subcutaneous treatment	ND	50	Viable tissue
5	Poorly differentiated lung cancer	ND	FNAB of inguinal lymph node	ND	100	Necrotic tissue
8	Poorly differentiated lung cancer	ND	FNAB of chest wall	ND	200	Necrotic tissue
9	Adenocarcinoma of lung	ND	ExB of supraclavicular lymph node	ND	200	Viable tissue
10	Squamous cell carcinoma of the lung	Bronchoscopic biopsy	Bronchoscopic biopsy	ND	400	Viable tissue
12	Adenocarcinoma of lung	ExB of subcutaneous met	ExB of subscutaneous mets		400	Viable tissue
13	Adenocarcinoma of lung	FNAB of supraclavicular node	ExB of supraclavicular node	ND	600	Viable tissue
14	Squamous carcinoma of tongue	Surgical Bx of neck tumor	Surgical Bx of neck tumor	Surgical Bx of neck tumor on day 9	600	Viable tissue
15	Squamous carcioma of larynxe	Surgical Bx of neck tumor	Surgical Bx of neck tumor	ND	600	Viable tissu

ND, not done; FNAB, fine needle aspiration and biopsy; ExB, excisional biopsy; Bx, biopsy. (From Perez-Soler et al. 1994)

Table 2. Image analysis of EGFR expression before and after RG 83852

| Patient no. | Total dose (mg/mg^2) | Intensity of EGFR expression[a] | | | | | |
| | | Pretreatment | | 6-day posttreatment | | 9-day posttreatment | |
		2° Ab[b]	1°+2° Ab[b]	2° Ab[b]	1°+2° Ab[b]	2° Ab[b]	1°+2° Ab[b]
2[c]	50	–	0.03	–	0.06	ND	
3	50	–	0.02	–	0.04	ND	
9[c]	200	–	0.05	–	0.09	ND	
10	400	–	0.09	0.05	0.14	ND	
12	400	–	0.05	0.02	0.04	ND	
14	600	–	0.16	0.07	0.23	0.03	0.19
15	600	–	0.19	0.08	0.14	ND	

[a]Intensity of EGFR expression measured by image analysis was normalized by 886 cells which were attached to each slide.
[b]2° Ab, secondary antibody; 1°+2° Ab, primary and secondary antibodies.
[c]Tumor tissue samples taken at initial diagnosis were used as pretreatment specimens.

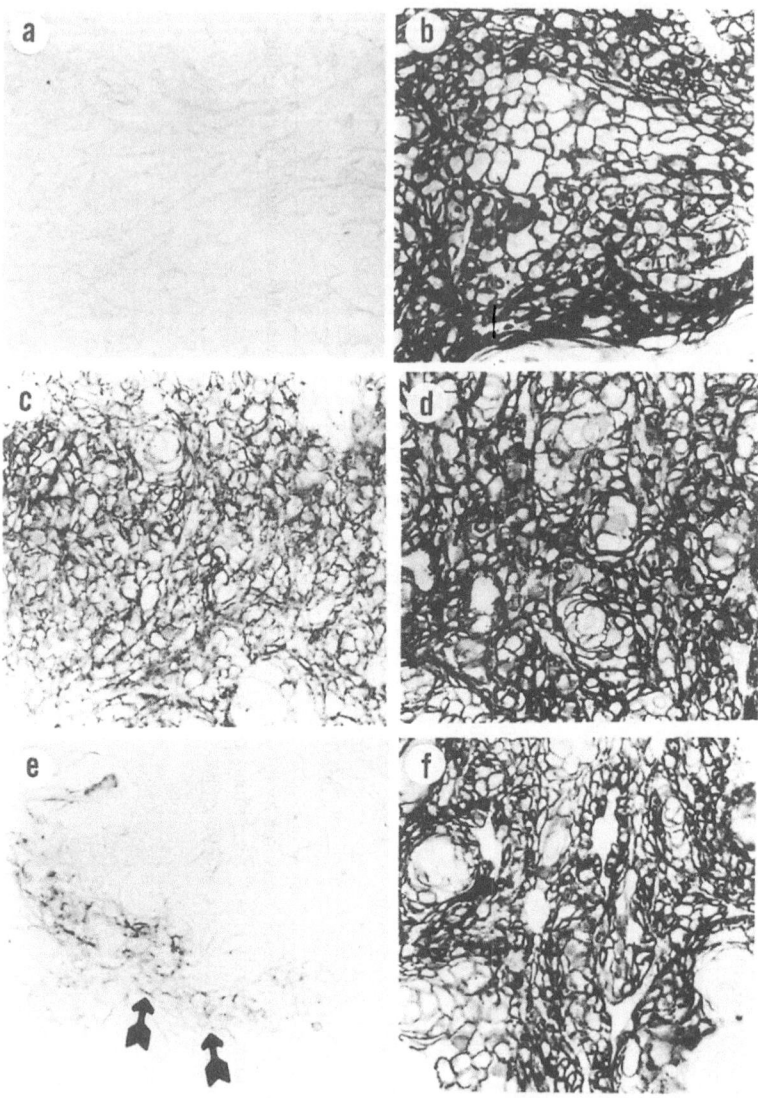

Fig. 1. Legend see p. 77

Immunohistochemical analysis was performed on paraffin-embedded tissue sections obtained from seven patients (Nos. 2, 3, 9, 10, 12, 14, and 15) by using a different monoclonal anti-EGFR antibody (BioGenex, Inc., San Ramon, CA, USA), because RG83852 reacts only with fresh tissue. The doses of RG83852 were 50 mg/m^2 in patient 2, 200 mg/m^2 in patient 9, 400 mg/m^2 in patients 10 and 12, and 600 mg/m^2 in patients 14 and 15. Immunohistochemical staining was applied on deparaffinized tissue sections as described elsewhere (Gown and Vogel 1984). In brief, after an initial blockade with nonimmune horse serum, the sections were incubated sequentially with the anti-EGFR antibody for 2 h at 37°C, biotinylated secondary antibody, and avidin–biotin–peroxidase conjugate solution (ABC) and were incubated with the peroxidase substitute 0.1% diaminobenzidine (DAB) in H_2O_2. For the purpose of assessing tumor EGFR saturation after RG83852 infusion, immunohistochemical staining using only secondary antibody was performed and compared with that of the sections incubated with anti-EGFR plus secondary antibodies. The degree of EGFR antibody was quantitated with the image analysis system as described earlier (Shin et al. 1994c).

Among 15 patients treated with RG83852, 13 had non-small-cell lung cancer and two had squamous cell carcinoma of the head and neck. Fourteen patients had received chemotherapy and/or radiotherapy. A total of 19 courses of RG83852 were administered (Table 1); 11 received a single course and four received two courses. Side effects were minimal; only one patient developed skin rashes, which responded to antihistamines. No other toxic effects were observed. No major tumor

◄ **Fig. 1a–f.** Immunohistochemical staining of epidermal growth factor receptor (EGFR) expression in the tumor of patient 14, who received RG83852 at 600 mg/m^2. **a,b** EGFR expression before infusion of RG83852 (at baseline): did not express EGFR when infused with secondary antibody alone (**a**); expressed EGFR at high levels when infused with primary and secondary antibodies (**b**). **c,d** EGFR expression on day 6 after 5 days of treatment with RG83852: expressed EGFR at moderate levels when infused with secondary antibody alone (**c**); expressed EGFR at high levels when infused with primary and secondary antibodies (**d**). **e,f** EGFR expression on day 9 after 5 days of treatment with RG83852: expressed EGFR at a low level (indicated by *arrows*) when infused with secondary antibody alone (**e**); expressed EGFR at a very high level when infused with both primary and secondary antibodies (**f**)

response at the clinical level was observed, except one patient with adenocarcinoma of the lung had softening of a tumor-involved lymph node.

The results of immunohistochemical staining of paraffin-embedded pretreatment and posttreatment specimens from seven patients (Nos. 2, 3, 9, 10, 12, 14, and 15) and initial tumor biopsies from two patients (Nos. 2 and 9) are shown in Table 2. Tumor EGFR saturation of RG83852 was observed in patients treated with a total dose of at least 400 mg/m^2 after the posttreatment tumor specimens were incubated with secondary antibody only. The degree of saturation was assessed quantitatively by image analysis. The intensity of the EGFR expression of the posttreament samples exposed to secondary antibody alone was compared with that of specimens exposed to both primary and secondary antibodies. A high degree of saturation was observed in patients 14 and 15, who received 600 mg/m^2 of RG83852. Upregulation of EGFR was observed in five of seven samples (Nos. 2, 3, 9, 10, and 14) by comparing intensity of staining in the pretreatment and posttreatment tumor specimens exposed to both primary and secondary antibodies. However, one sample showed slight downregulation of EGFR (No. 15) and another did not demonstrate any change (No. 12).

Figure 1 demonstrates the immunostaining for EGFR expression in patient 14, in Fig. 1a,b at baseline, in parts c,d on day 6 after 5 days of treatment with GR83852, and in parts e,f on day 9 after 5 days of treatment. The intensities of EGFR expression in Fig. 1a,c,e were 0, 0.07, and 0.03, respectively, representing samples incubated with secondary antibody alone. The intensities of EGFR expression of Fig. 1b,d,f were 0.16, 0.23, and 0.19, representing samples incubated with both primary and secondary antibodies. In the day-6 sample from patient 14 (Fig. 1c), a significant amount of RG83852 bound to the tumor specimen was localized by secondary antibody alone, and the intensity of expression was further increased to 0.23 after incubation with both primary and secondary antibodies. In this particular case, we were able to obtain a day-9 posttreatment sample, which showed a small amount of RG83852 still bound to the tumor tissue, as shown in Fig. 1e.

4.6 Discussion

The purpose of this study was to better understand the role of EGFR
expression in aerodigestive tract tumorigenesis and its therapeutic implications in the clinical setting. A variety of clinical evidence, including
studies in oral leukoplakia, had indicated that head and neck tumor
development involved a multistep process occurring in a field repeatedly
exposed to carcinogens. In a hamster buccal pouch tumor model, we and
others demonstrated that EGFR expression increased in a multistep
fashion during tumorigenesis (Shin et al. 1994a; Wong and Biswas
1986; Wong 1987). In particular, premalignant lesions (i.e., hyperplasia
and dysplasia) had high EGFR expression at the protein level in our
study (Shin et al. 1994a) and at the mRNA level in studies by others
(Wong and Biswas 1986), suggesting that EGFR expression may play
an important role in transformation from normal through premalignant
changes to squamous cell carcinoma. Micronuclei frequency was assessed for the measure of nuclei aberration responsive to the genotoxic-
ity of DMBA in the buccal pouch of hamsters. The micronuclei frequency was highly elevated in hyperplasia and dysplasia and correlated
with the increased level of EGFR expression. This finding suggests that
genomic instability is ongoing in premalignant tissue in this animal
model.

The prematurely condensed chromosome (PCC) technique was used
to determine chromosomal aberrations associated with the carcinogenesis process in the hamster buccal pouch model. This analysis revealed
two important findings (Hittelman et al. 1991). First, numerical chromosome changes were observed in the hyperplastic lesions derived from
tissues treated for 4 weeks with DMBA and were observed to accumulate with continued carcinogen exposure. Second, chromosomal damage
was observed through the field of exposure, not only in the specific sites
in which tumors ultimately developed. This illustrates the notion of
"field cancerization," whereby a whole tissue exposed to a carcinogen is
at increased risk for the development of tumors.

In our study of tumorigenesis in human head and neck cancer, we
used tumor tissue specimens that contained adjacent normal tissue,
hyperplastic lesions, and/or dysplastic lesions and found that upregulation of EGFR expression occurred in two stages; the first change occurred between normal control epithelium derived from nonsmokers

and normal epithelium adjacent to tumors, and the second with the transition from dysplastic lesions to squamous cell carcinomas. EGFR expression in histologically normal-appearing epithelium adjacent to the tumors was twice as high as in the control epithelium of individuals who were never exposed to smoking or alcohol. These findings support the field cancerization and multistep nature of the tumorigenesis process that has been demonstrated in the hamster buccal pouch model. Therefore, the increased expression of EGFR in the normal adjacent epithelial tissue may be a result of factors expressed by the tumors that cause phenotypic and other genetic changes in this biologically dynamic tissue field.

On the adjacent sections of the same tissue specimens, we analyzed PCNA expression by immunohistochemical analysis (Shin et al. 1993). PCNA expression increased threefold from the normal control epithelia to the adjacent normal epithelial tissue. The high PCNA expression in the normal tissue adjacent to tumor suggests that the carcinogen-exposed field has a much higher proliferative potential than control epithelia never exposed to carcinogens even in the same histologically normal tissue. Therefore, EGFR dysregulation and PCNA expression might be useful markers for characterizing the degree of proliferative dysregulation, whereby an entire carcinogen-exposed tissue field is at increased risk for developing multiple, independent foci of tumor development. At the clinical level, these multiple tumors can occur at the same time or at different times in the aerodigestive tract (Auerbach et al. 1957; Gluckman et al. 1980; Shibuya et al. 1987; Snow et al. 1987). This clinical observation supports the notion that the carcinogen-exposed tissue represents a field at increased risk for tumor development.

The proliferative dysregulation is continuously increased through the progression from premalignant lesions (i.e., hyperplasia, dysplasia) to squamous cell carcinomas. Dysplastic lesions, in particular, had nearly the same degree of proliferative activity as the tumor region, suggesting that some of the genetic alterations may have occurred prior to tumor development. To visualize the accumulation of genetic alterations during head and neck tumorigenesis, and to determine the extent of the genetically altered field, we studied chromosome abnormalities in squamous cell carcinomas of the head and neck and in their adjacent premalignant lesions. Using chromosome specific probes for chromosomes 7 and 17, nonradioactive in situ hybridization was applied to the paraffin-embedded tissue sections (Voravud et al. 1993). Normal oral epithelium from cancer-free nonsmokers showed no chromosome polysomy (i.e., cells with three or more chromosome copies per cell), whereas histologically normal epithelium adjacent to tumors showed multiple copies of chromosome 7 or 17. Furthermore, the frequency of cells with polysomy increased as the tissues progressed to hyperplasia, to dysplasia, and to cancer. These findings clearly support the concept that increased dysregulation of proliferative activity in the carcinogen-exposed field is associated with genetic instability during the process of tumor formation. This biomarker study will be an important tool in chemoprevention and therapeutic trials (Lippman et al. 1990; Shin et al. 1994b; Shin et al. 1996).

The last part of our study was concerned with whether EGFR antibodies reach the tumor in significant amounts during the intravenous administration of anti-EGFR monoclonal antibody RG83852. We used two different methods to evaluate tumor EGFR saturation with the antibody. The tyrosine kinase activity of EGFR-RG83852 complexes obtained from fresh tissue homogenates was measured by immunoprecipitation in the presence or absence of an exogenous saturating concentration of RG83852 (Perez-Soler et al. 1994). With this technique, we observed partial tumor saturation (80%) in a patient who received 200 mg/m^2 of RG83852, 50% in a patient who received 400 mg/m^2, and 100% in two of three patients who received 600 mg/m^2. By standard immunohistochemical methods for paraffin-embedded tissue, we observed tumor localization of RG83852 in patients treated with doses greater than 400 mg/m^2 but no tumor localization of RG83852 in patients who received 200 mg/m^2. Full tumor saturation was observed in patients who were treated with 600 mg/m^2. The discrepancy may be attributed to the fact that RG83852 and the antibody used for the immunohistochemical study recognize different epitopes on EGFR. The most important finding in this study was the upregulation of tumor EGFR expression and tyrosine kinase activity when we infused RG83852 to the patients. This observation may be shown to have important therapeutic implications in future studies.

A study from Sturgis et al. (1994) showed that anti-EGFR antibody 528 inhibited the growth of monolayer head and neck cells bearing high levels of EGFR and promoted differentiation in some tumor cells. External beam irradiation has been shown to enhance accumulation of monoclonal antibodies in tumors in vivo. Bender et al. (1995) tested high-grade glioma cell lines U87-MG and A1207 with the ^{125}I-labeled monoclonal antibody 425 that binds specifically to the human EGFR. Irradiation of high-grade glioma cells markedly enhanced the binding of ^{125}I-labeled monoclonal antibody 425 to the cell surface. At the same time, irradiation stimulated significant and dose-dependent internalization of this antibody. Bender et al. concluded that the combination of external beam irradiation and labeled monoclonal antibody 425 showed at least additive effects on the radiocytotoxicity.

The same monoclonal antibody, 425, was given to 59 patients with high-grade gliomas in an adjuvant setting (Snelling et al. 1995). Total cumulative, labeled antibody doses ranging from 40 to 296 mCi were administered to the patients within 3 months following completion of surgery and postoperative radiation therapy. No significant toxic effects were observed. One year after treatment, 34 of the 59 patients (58%) in this trial were alive. In addition, sensitivity to cisplatin has been shown to correlate with the amount of EGFR expression in a panel of cervical squamous carcinoma cell lines (Nishikawa et al. 1992). This study suggests that sensitivity to cisplatin may be potentiated by stimulation of EGFR tyrosine kinase activity and may correlate with the level of transmembrane tyrosine kinase activity within the cells.

Since our study results indicate that both EGFR tyrosine kinase activity and EGFR expression were markedly enhanced 24 h after the administration of RG83852, it is conceivable that such an increase may be associated with an enhanced sensitivity to cisplatin in the subset of patients with cancers of the head and neck. Most of the hyperplastic or dysplastic lesions in these patients also had high EGFR expression. Therefore, to inhibit further progression to the tumors, monoclonal anti-EGFR antibody therapy with or without other differentiating agents may be considered for these premalignant lesions in future chemoprevention trials.

Acknowledgment. We wish to thank Trupti Shah for skillful technical assistance, Maria J. Scliris for the preparation of the manuscript, and Kathryn Hale for editorial assistance.

References

Aboud-Pirak E, Hurwitz E, Pirak ME et al. (1988) Efficacy of antibodies to epidermal growth factor receptor against KB carcinoma in vitro and in nude mice. J Natl Cancer Inst 80:1605–1611

Aboud-Pirak E, Hurwitz E, Bellot F et al. (1989) Inhibition of human tumor growth in nude mice elicited by monoclonal anti-EGF receptor antibodies conjugated with doxorubicin. Proc Natl Acad Sci USA 86:3777–3781

Auerbach O, Gere B, Forman JB et al. (1957) Changes in the bronchial epithelium in relation to cigarette smoking and cancer of the lung. N Engl J Med 256:97–104

Auerbach O, Stout AP, Hammond EC, Garfinkel L (1961) Changes in bronchial epithelium in relation to cigarette smoking and in relation to lung cancer. N Engl J Med 265:253–267

Bender H, Emrich JG, Eshelman J, Chu MA, Steplewski Z, Biersack HJ, Brady LW (1995) Enhancement of monoclonal antibody efficacy: the effect of external beam radiation. Hybridoma 14:129–134

Cerny T, Barnes DM, Hasleton P, Baber PV, Healey K, Gullick W, Thatcher N (1986) Expression of epidermal growth factor receptor (EGF-r) in human lung tumors. Br J Cancer 54:265–269

Christen RD, Hom DK, Porter DC et al. (1990) Epidermal growth factor regulates the in vitro sensitivity of human ovarian carcinoma cells to cisplatin. J Clin Invest 86:1632–1640

Cohen S, Carpenter G, King L (1980) Epithelial growth factor receptor protein kinase interactions. J Biol Chem 255:4834–4842

Cohen S, Ushiro H, Stoscheck C, Gill GN (1985) Regulation of the epidermal growth factor by phosphorylation. J Cell Biochem 29:195–208

Derynek R (1988) Transforming growth factor-α. Cell 54:593–595

Divigi CR, Welt S, Kris M et al. (1991) Phase I and imaging trial of indium 111-labeled anti-epidermal growth factor receptor monoclonal antibody 225 in patients with squamous cell lung carcinoma. J Natl Cancer Inst 83:97–104

Eisbruch A, Blick M, Lee JS, Sacks PG, Gutterman J (1987) Analysis of the epidermal growth factor receptor gene in fresh human head and neck tumors. Cancer Res 47:3603–3605

Farber E (1984) The multistep nature of cancer development. Cancer Res 44:4217–4223

Filmus J, Pollack MN, Cailleau R, Buick RM (1985) MDA-468, a human breast cancer cell line with a high number of epidermal growth factor (EGF) receptors, has an amplified EGF receptor gene and is growth inhibited by EGF. Biochem Biophys Res Commun 128:898–905

Gill GN, Kawamoto T, Cochet C et al. (1984) Monoclonal anti-epidermal growth factor receptor (EGFR) antibodies which are inhibitors of EGF binding and antagonists of EGF-stimulated tyrosine protein kinase activity. J Biol Chem 259:7755–7760

Gluckman JL, Crissman JD, Donegan JO (1980) Multicenter squamous cell carcinoma of the upper aerodigestive tract. Head Neck Surg 3:90–96

Gown AM, Vogel AM (1984) Monoclonal antibodies to human intermediate filament protein II. Distribution of filament proteins in normal tissues. Am J Pathol 114:309–321

Gusterson B, Cowley G, Smith JA, Ozanne B (1984) Cellular localization of human epidermal growth factor receptor. Cell Biol Int Rep 8:649–657

Hendler FJ, Ozanne BW (1984) Human squamous cell lung cancers express increase of epidermal growth factor receptors. J Clin Invest 74:647–651

Hittelman WN, Lee JS, Cheong N, Shin DM, Hong WK (1991) The chromosome view of "field cancerization" and multistep carcinogenesis. Implication for chemopreventive approaches. In: Pastorino U, Hong WK (eds) Chemoimmunoprevention of cancer. Thieme, Stuttgart, pp 41–47

Hong WK, Lippman SM, Itr LM et al. (1990) Prevention of second primary tumors with isotretinoin in squamous cell carcinoma of the head and neck. N Engl J Med 323:795–801

Jaskulski D, DeRiel JK, Mercer WE et al. (1988) Inhibition of cellular proliferation by antisense oligodeoxynucleotides to PCNA cyclin. Science 240:1544–1546

Kwok TT, Sutherland RM (1989) Enhancement of sensitivity of human squamous cells to radiation by epidermal growth factor receptor. J Natl Cancer Inst 81:1020–1024

Kwok TT, Sutherland RM (1991) Differences in EGFR related radiosensitization of human squamous cells with high and low numbers of EGF receptors. Br J Cancer 64:251–254

Lax I, Bellot F, Howk R, Ullirich A et al. (1989) Functional analysis of the ligand binding site of EGFR-receptor utilizing chimeric chicken/human receptor molecules. EMBO J 8:421–427

Libermann TA, Nusbaum HR, Razon N et al. (1985). Amplification, enhanced expression and possible rearrangement of EGFR gene in primary human brain tumors of glial origin. Nature 313:144–147

Lippman SM, Hong WK (1989) Second malignant tumors in head and neck squamous cell carcinoma: the overshadowing threat for patients with early-stage disease. Int J Radiat Oncol Biol Phys 17:691–694

Lippman SM, Lee JS, Lotan R et al. (1990) Biomarkers as intermediate end points in chemoprevention trials. J Natl Cancer Inst 82:555–560

Lippman SM, Benner SE, Hong WK (1994). Cancer chemoprevention. J Clin Oncol 12:851–873

Masui H, Kawamoto T, Sato JD et al. (1984) Growth inhibition of human tumor cells in athymic nude mice by anti-epidermal growth factor receptor monoclonal antibodies. Cancer Res 44:1002–1007

Maxwell SA, Sacks PG, Gutterman JU, Gallick GE (1989) Epidermal growth factor receptor protein-tyrosine kinase activity in human cell lines established from squamous carcinomas of the head and neck. Cancer Res 49:1130–1137

Meyskens FL Jr (1990) Coming of age: the chemoprevention of cancer. N Engl J Med 323:825–827

Morris AL (1961) Factors influencing experimental carcinogenesis in the hamster cheek pouch. J Dent Res 40:3–15

Nishikawa K, Rosenblum MG, Newman R et al. (1992) Resistance of human cervical carcinoma cells to tumor necrosis factor correlates with their increased sensitivity to cisplatin: evidence of a role for DNA repair and epidermal growth factor receptor. Cancer Res 52:4758–4765

Ozanne B, Richards CS, Hendler F, Burns D, Gusterson B (1986) Overexpression of the EGF receptor is a hallmark of squamous cell carcinomas. J Pathol 149:9–14

Perez-Soler R, Donato NJ, Shin DM et al. (1994) Tumor epidermal growth factor receptor studies in patients with non-small-cell lung cancer or head and neck cancer treated with monoclonal antibody RG83852. J Clin Oncol 12:730–739

Salley JJ (1954) Experimental carcinogenesis in the cheek pouch of the Syrian hamster. J Dent Res 33:253–262

Salley JJ (1957) Histologic changes in the hamster cheek pouch during early hydrocarbon carcinogenesis. J Dent Res 36:48–55

Santini J, Formento JL, Francoval M, Milano G, Schneider M, Dassonville O, Dernard F (1991) Characterization, quantitation and potential clinical value of the epidermal growth factor receptor in head and neck squamous cell carcinomas. Head Neck 13:132–139

Schwartz J, Shklar G (1988) Regression of experimental oral carcinogenesis by local injection of beta-carotene and camthoxanthine. Nutr Cancer 11:35–40

Schwartz J, Shklar G, Reid S, Trickler D (1988) Prevention of oral cancer by extracts of Spirulina-Dunaliella algae. Nutr Cancer 11:127–134

Shibuya H, Hisamitsu S, Shioiri S et al. (1987) Multiple primary cancer risk in patients with squamous cell carcinoma of the oral cavity. Cancer 60:3083–3086

Shin DM, Voravud N, Ro JY, Lee JS, Hong WK, Hittelman WN (1993) Sequential increase of proliferating cell nuclear antigen (PCNA) in head and neck carcinogenesis: a potential biomarker. J Natl Cancer Inst 85:971–977

Shin DM, Gimenez IB, Lee JS et al. (1994a) Expression of epidermal growth factor receptor, polyamine levels, ornithine decarboxylase activity, micronuclei, and transglutaminase I in a 7, 12-dimethylbenz (a) anthracene-induced hamster buccal pouch carcinogenesis model. Cancer Res 50:2505–2510

Shin DM, Hittelman WN, Hong WK (1994b) Biomarkers in upper aerodigestive tract tumorigenesis: a review. Cancer Epidermal Biomarkers Prev 3:697–709

Shin DM, Ro JY, Hong WK, Hittelman WN (1994c) Dysregulation of epidermal growth factor receptor expression in premalignant lesions during head and neck tumorigenesis. Cancer Res 54:3153–3159

Shin DM, Lee JS, Lippman SM et al. (1996) p53 expression: predicting recurrence and second primary tumors in head and neck squamous cell carcinoma. J Natl Cancer Inst 88:519–529

Shklar G (1965) Metabolic characteristics of experimental hamster pouch carcinomas. Oral Surg 20:336–339

Shklar G (1982) Oral mucosal carcinogenesis in hamster: inhibition by vitamin E. J Natl Cancer Inst 68:791–799

Silverman S, Shklar G (1963). The effect of a carcinogen (DMBA) applied to the hamster cheek pouch in combination with croton oil. Oral Surg 16:1344–1355

Silverman SJ Jr., Gorsky M, Lozada F (1984) Oral leukoplakia and malignant transformation: a follow-up study of 257 patients. Cancer 53:563–568

Slaughter DL, Southwick HW, Smejkal W (1953) "Field cancerization" in oral stratified squamous epithelium: clinical implications of multicentric origin. Cancer 6:963–968

Snelling L, Miyamoto CT, Bender H, Brady LW et al. (1995) Epidermal growth factor receptor 425 monoclonal antibodies radiolabeled with iodine-125 in the adjuvant treatment of high-grade astrocytomas. Hybridoma 14:111–114

Snow GB, De Vries N, Van Zandwijk N et al. (1987) Secondary primary cancers in the lung and head and neck cancer patients: a challenge. Eur J Cancer Clin Oncol 23:883–886

Sturgis EM, Sacks PG, Masui H, Mendelsohn J, Schantz SP (1994) Effects of antiepidermal growth factor receptor antibody 528 on the proliferation and differentiation of head and neck cancer. Otolaryngol Head Neck Surg 111:633–643

Suda D, Schwartz J, Shklar G (1986). Inhibition of experimental oral carcinogenesis by topical beta-carotene. Carcinogenesis 7:711–715

Todd R, Donoff BR, Gertz R et al. (1989) TGF-α and EGF receptor mRNAs in human oral cancers. Carcinogenesis 10:1553–1556

Trickler D, Shklar G (1987) Prevention by vitamin E of experimental oral carcinogenesis. J Natl Cancer Inst 78:165–169

Tsiklakis K, Papadakou A, Angelopoulos AP (1987) The therapeutic effects of an aromatic retinoid (R0-109359) on hamster buccal pouch carcinomas. Oral Surg 64:327–332

Ushiro H, Cohen S (1980) Identification of phosphotyrosine as a product of epidermal growth factor-activated protein kinase in A431 cell membranes. J Biol Chem 255:8363–8365

Velu TJ, Beguinot L, Vass WC, Willingham MC, Merlino GT, Pastan I, Lowy DR (1987) Epidermal growth factor dependent transformation by a human EGF receptor protooncogene. Science 238:1408–1410

Voravud N, Shin DM, Ro JY, Lee JS, Hong WK, Hittelman WN (1993) Increased polysomies of chromosomes 7 and 17 during head and neck multistep tumorigenesis. Cancer Res 53:2874–2883

Weichselbaum RR, Dunphy EJ, Beckett MA et al. (1989) Epidermal growth factor receptor gene amplification and expression in head and neck cancer cell lines. Head Neck 11:437–442

Wong DTW (1987) Amplification of the C-erbBI oncogene in chemically induced oral carcinomas. Carcinogenesis 8:1963–1965

Wong DTW, Biswas DK (1986) Activation of the C-erbB oncogene during DMBA-induced carcinogenesis in hamster cheek pouch. J Dent Res 65:221

Yamamoto T, Nishida T, Miyajima M, Kawai S, Ooi T, Toyoshima K (1983) The erbB gene of the avian erythroblastosis virus is a member of the Src gene family. Cell 35:71–78

5 EGF Receptors as a Target for Therapy and Interactions with Angiogenesis

A.L. Harris

5.1 Introduction

The epidermal growth factor receptor (EGFR) is a transmembrane tyrosine kinase activated by several ligands besides EGF. Its expression in normal tissues and cancer has been extensively studied by immunohistochemistry and ligand-binding assays. Since it was found to be a transforming gene in vitro and in vivo assays and commonly unregulated in cancer with a poor prognosis, its potential as a therapy target has been investigated and clinical trials are now in progress. This article reviews the clinical background and some recent developments with implications for therapy.

5.2 The EGFR and Prognosis

The EGFR was the first receptor tyrosine kinase in its class, but several more are now known, including c-erbB-2, erbB-3 and erbB-4. These receptors may heterodimerise to produce higher affinity receptors (Earp et al. 1995). This is the case for erbB-2, which is commonly amplified in breast cancer and associated with poor prognosis and poor response to chemotherapy and hormone therapy (Wright et al. 1992a,b). Cases with high EGFR and high c-erbB-2 have a particularly poor prognosis (Wright et al. 1989). In many common epithelial neoplasms, tumours with high EGFR compared to the median level in tumours or normal tissues have a worse prognosis (reviewed in Harris 1990, 1991). This has been extensively investigated in breast cancer, where EGFr expression is inversely related to oestrogen receptor (ER). Over 10 000 cases have been reported in various studies, and although some studies do not confirm poor prognosis, the majority do (Fox et al. 1994b; Klijn et al. 1992). High EGFR is associated with resistance to hormone therapy (Nicholson et al. 1988, 1989).

One of the problems in investigating any new pathway in human tumour biology is tissue collection, extraction and methodology of assays, which are hardly ever standardised, except in the case of the ER. This needs to be taken into account when selecting patients for multicentre trials of new therapy approaches. We recently showed that there is a good correlation of antibody staining on paraffin sections with ligand-binding assays for EGFR in breast cancer (Newby et al. 1995).

EGFR expression has also been associated with a high frequency of recurrence of bladder cancer (Neal et al. 1985) and progression to a more invasive phenotype (Neal et al. 1990), and poor survival after surgery for non-small-cell lung cancer (Veale et al. 1993). In the latter tumour type, EGFR may be expressed at levels greater than 100-fold higher than in normal lung tissue (Veale et al. 1989). Amplification of the EGFR is found in the most aggressive types of gliomasglioblastoma multiforms and there may also be rearrangements of the sequences coding for the extracellular, ligand-binding site of the receptor (Schober et al. 1995; Rao et al. 1996).

5.3 EGFR and Tumour Angiogenesis

In most squamous cancers, including vulva, cervix, oesophagus and head and neck cancer, there is high expression of EGFR. The effect of high angiogenesis in patients with high EGFR in their breast cancers has recently been studied (Fox et al. 1994a). Angiogenesis is critical for growth and metastasis of tumours and in some human tumour cell lines in vitro EGF stimulates the production of the specific endothelial mitogen vascular endothelial cell growth factor (VEGF). Thus, EGF may have a paracrine effect on angiogenesis. We assessed this interaction in breast cancer. We used a monoclonal antibody to the endothelial cell adhesion molecule CD31 to stain tumour blood vessels and quantitatively assessed vascular density (Horak et al. 1992). Vascular density was also assessed using a Chalkley eye-piece to achieve better quantification. High vascular density has been shown in many studies to be related to poor prognosis. In a series of 109 node-negative patients, high

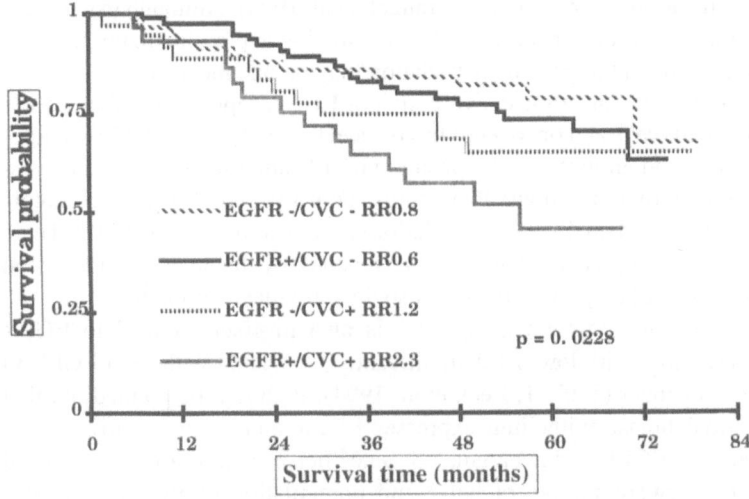

Fig. 1. Epidermal growth factor receptor (*EGFR*) and angiogenesis in prognosis. EGFR-positive cases are those with 20 fmol/mg membrane protein or greater. Chalkley vessel counts (*CVC*) are stratified into an upper third and lower two thirds, CVC+ being the upper third. *RR*, relative risk of relapse

vascular density predicted for poor overall and relapse-free survival. Although high EGFR was associated with poor survival if stratified by vascular density (VD), it was only those patients with high VD who had poor survival, and those patients with high EGFR with low VD had similar survival to those who were EGFR negative. This result was also found in a combined series of over 200 patients, including node-positive patients and the node-negative patients described above (Fig. 1). Thus, therapy approaches blocking both angiogenesis and EGFR should be considered.

5.4 Mechanisms of Upregulation of EGFR

Although gene amplification is a common mechanism of upregulation of c-erbB-2 in breast cancer, EGFR is rarely amplified in breast cancer (3% of cases). Nevertheless, similar levels of expression of EGFR can occur with or without amplification. High levels of mRNA are associated with high EGFR so mechanisms of transcription regulation or stabilisation are important (Petrangeli et al. 1995). Although extensively studied, as yet no specific factor-upregulating expression in tumours has been defined but gene demethylation may be one mechanism.

In breast cancer the coexpression of EGF receptor with other signalling pathways and oncogenes has been extensively studied. Most studies have found an inverse relationship with ER and this is the most consistent pattern. On tumours that express both ER and EGFR the receptors are expressed on different populations (van Agthoven et al. 1995). There may be reciprocal regulation of one receptor by the other and it has been shown that heregulin (HR) can also downregulate ER expression.

The anti-apoptotic gene bcl-2 is also inversely related to EGFR expression, with low bcl-2 significantly associated with high EGFR in breast cancer (Table 1; Leek et al. 1994). It should be pointed out that normal breast epithelium expresses EGFR and in ER-positive breast cancers, EGFR is downregulated. Since bcl-2 is an oestrogen-regulated gene, downregulation of bcl-2 and upregulation of EGFR may both reflect a loss of ER function and therefore also hormone resistance.

There are several types of mutations involving the external ligand-binding domain of the EGFR, particularly in gliomas. These result in a constitutively activated receptor and would not be detected by conven-

Table 1. EGFR and bcl-2 expression in breast cancer

	bcl-2-positive Invasive tumours	bcl-2-negative Invasive tumours	p Value
ER positive	70	7	
ER negative	18	16	
ER positive (%)	80	30	<0.0001
EGFR positive	26	16	
EGFR negative	62	7	
EGRF positive (%)	30	70	0.001
c-erb-B-2 positive	2	6	
c-erb-B-2 negative	49	13	
c-erb-B-2 positive (%)	4	32	0.004
p53 positive	27	15	
p53 negative	52	6	
p53 positive	34	71	0.005

ER, oestrogen receptor; EGFR, epidermal growth factor receptor.

tional ligand-binding assays or antibodies that react with the external domain. Because a new peptide sequence is generated by the deletions, antibodies to these have been developed for specific staining of mutated EGFR (Wikstrand et al. 1995). There is evidence that these aberrant receptors may also be present in two much commoner tumour types, breast and non-small-cell lung cancer. Since these aberrant receptors are tumour specific, mutant extracellular domains they provide an attractive target for therapy.

5.5 Novel EGFR Ligands and Their Sources in Human Tumours

EGF and transforming growth factor-α (TGF-α) were the original ligands found for the EGFR, as well as various viral proteins with EGF-like domains. Several other ligands expressed in tumours and normal tissues have been described, including amphiregulin (AR; Lejeune et al. 1993), betacellulin, heparin-binding EGF and epiregulin (Toyoda et al. 1995; Groenen et al. 1994). Because the nonmutated EGFR requires a ligand for transforming activity, it is likely that the levels of expression

Table 2. EGF family ligands: relationship between amphiregulin+, heregulin+ and cripto -1+ mRNA – EGFR and c-erbB-2 in breast cancer

Receptor	Amphiregulin+ 35/60 (58)	Heregulin+ 15/60 (25)	Cripto -1+ 46/60 /72)
EGFr+ 46/60 (77)	25/46 (54)	10/46 (22)	34/46 (74)
erbB-2+ 12/41 (29)	7/12 (58)	1/12 (8)	7/12 (58)
ER+ 51/60 (85)	35/51 (69)*	11/51 (22)	39/51 (76)

Numbers in parentheses indicate % positive at mRNA analysis.
EGFR, epidermal growth factor receptor; ER, oestrogen receptor.

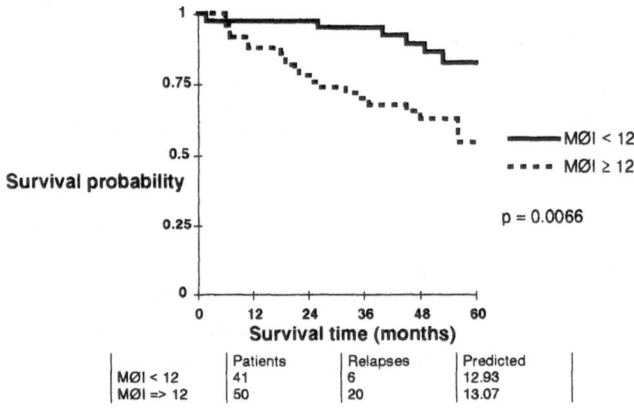

Hazard Ratio = 3.32   95% CI = 1.33,8.27   Chi Squared = 7.39   p = 0.0066

Fig. 2. Relapse-free survival in breast cancer, stratified by macrophage counts. Macrophages were stained with an antibody to CD68 and counted using a Chalkley eye-piece. Results are stratified by the median count

of these ligands may also be relevant to tumour behaviour and prognosis (Saeki et al. 1995; Lupu et al. 1995). In many tumour types, TGF-α is upregulated and expressed by tumour cells, providing both an autocrine and paracrine loop (Scher et al. 1995). We studied the coexpression of several of these ligands (60 breast cancers) and also the ligands associated with erbB-2 activation HR and found a complex pattern (Table 2).

Amphiregulin was expressed in approximately 60% of cases, HR in 25% and cripto-1 (CR-) in 77% as assessed by Northern blots and polymerase chain reaction (Normanno et al. 1995). There was no relationship of expression of the EGFR ligands amphiregulin or the erbB-2 heterodimer ligand HR to their respective receptors. In some 12% of cases none of the three ligands were expressed and in 55% two or more were expressed.

These studies are relevant to therapeutic strategies that involve targeting the ligand-binding domain of the EGFR, since high endogenous ligands may compete with targeting antibodies or fusion proteins involving EGF and TGF-α.

Although tumour cells produce many growth factors, approximately 50% of the cells in tumours are host nonmalignant cells which may also produce growth factors. We showed that human breast tumours contain macrophages that secrete EGF (O'Sullivan et al. 1993) and that the numbers of macrophages present in breast cancers are directly related to poor prognosis (Fig. 2). Thus, EGF may be contributing from this normal cellular population to tumour growth. Indeed, there is a strong correlation of EGFR expression in the primary tumours with macrophage numbers. Macrophages are also known to produce TGF-α but whether they make other ligands is not known.

5.6 Targeting EGFR

Monoclonal antibodies binding to the ligand-binding domain of EGFR have produced good localisation in xenografts with high EGFR (Goldstein et al. 1995), but because they have been human specific did not give a good guide to differential localisation. In patients, several studies have shown tumour selectivity, but there is also high uptake in the liver which expresses EGFR.

The use of antibodies to the mutated external domain is also planned if the expression of this type of receptor occurs in the more common solid tumours and is also planned for gliomas.

Because of high interstitial pressure in tumours and poor tissue penetration, several groups are investigating the use of stable scfv domains of EGFR antibodies and f(ab')(2) fragments (Tosi et al. 1995).

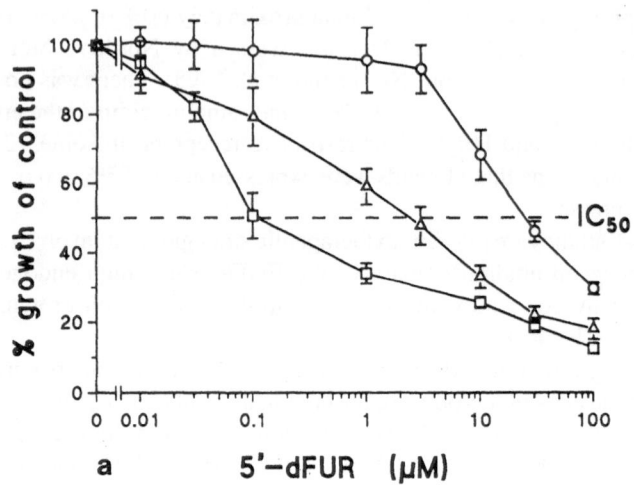

a   5'-dFUR (μM)

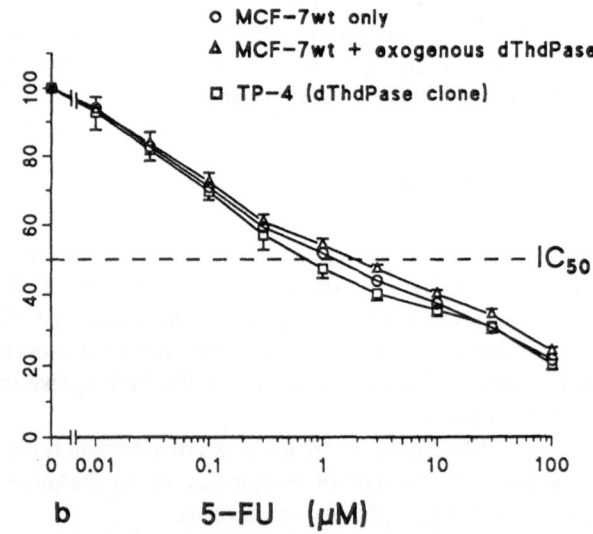

b   5-FU (μM)

Fig. 3. Legend see p. 97

Although they have better tissue penetration, they are also cleared more rapidly, so they may be better for imaging than therapy.

The use of antibodies includes delivering drugs, radiation or prodrug-activating enzymes. The last appears to be most likely to be effective since activating a much more readily diffusable prodrug overcomes the problem of tissue penetration and also heterogeneity of expression of the antigen. A problem with the activation enzymes is that most are nonhuman so antibodies may be made against them, reducing the ability to carry out repetitive dosing.

We therefore have investigated the use of human thymidine phosphorylase which can activate the 5-fluorouracil (5-FU) prodrug furtulon (Patterson et al. 1995). Overexpression of this gene intracellularly can produce over 100-fold sensitisation to furtulon and because no co-factors are required, the enzyme is equally effective if added extracellularly (Fig. 3). Since many tumours with high EGFR may be sensitive to 5-FU this may be of use in a broad spectrum of cancers (e.g. breast, colon, renal). Thymidine phosphorylase also degrades thymidine to thymine. This would deprive the thymidine salvage pathway and enhance the activity of drugs inhibiting de novo thymidine synthesis, e.g. methotrexate. Thus, this approach may also be of value in tumours with high EGFR that are treated with methotrexate (e.g. head and neck cancer, bladder and breast cancer).

Antibodies that block EGFR-binding EGF are synergistic with chemotherapy in in vivo models, including the drugs adriamycin and cis-platinum. The mechanism is not clear but may be via enhanced apoptosis and withdrawal of growth factors essential for survival after cytotoxic damage. This approach is now being studied in phase 1, using doses of EGFR-blocking antibodies that achieve levels in vivo known to inhibit EGF binding in vitro.

◀ **Fig. 3a,b.** Dose-response curves of MCF-7 carcinoma cell line to 5-fluououracil (5-FU, **b**) and its "prodrug" furtulon (5'-dFUR; **a**) in the presence of either intracellular or extracellular human thymidine phosphorylase. Exogenously added extracellular activity = 20.4 nmol dThd released per hour per milligram protein = 10^4 TP-4 cells = initial seeding density. * (*TP*) extracellularly activates furtulon (5=dFUR). There is no difference between the control cell lines, or cell line transfected with TP in 5FU sensitivity. Transfected or extracellular TP enhances furtulon activity

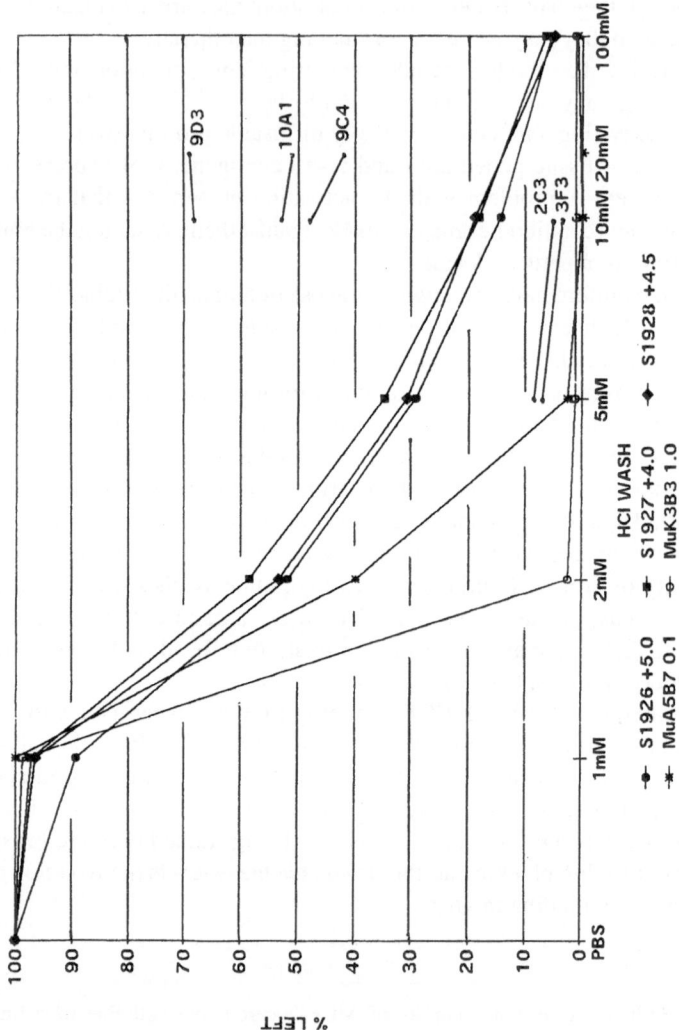

Fig. 4. High-affinity monoclonal antibody from sheep, binding to CEA. The resistance of sheep monoclonal antibodies to acid washes (ELISA) is shown. CEA is the antigen. Data provided by Dr. Peter Harrison of KS Biomedix Holdings plc, 212, Piccadilly, London WIV 9LD

EGF itself given with chemotherapy also enhances anticancer effects in vivo (Kroning et al. 1995). This may be due to the high doses given which may downregulate EGFR or by causing an increase in growth fraction-sensitive tumours to chemotherapy. Because of the high doses and short half-life, this is not likely to be useful clinically. However, it may be useful as a scanning agent when radiolabelled, because of its small size and, therefore, good tissue penetration (Cuarteroplaza et al. 1996).

In contrast, using EGFR ligands, modified such that they comprise a potent toxin such as diphtheria toxin or pseudomonas exotoxin has a better therapeutic effect (Fitzgerald and Pastan 1989). These proteins are smaller than antibodies and are internalised where they are potent inhibitors of protein synthesis. Intravesical therapy showed some antitumour effects in superficial bladder tumours, but the problem remains binding to enough tumour cells to produce a worthwhile response. Although there is a general correlation of high EGFR expression in cell lines with response to these toxins in vitro, there remains unexplained variation between them (Kirk et al. 1994). This may be due to subcellular localisation and compartmentalisation as well as differences in components of protein synthesis, e.g. concentrations of subunits. There is still the problem of having to target to each tumour cell, in contrast to the prodrug strategy.

Another way to exploit the tumour dependence of the EGFR pathway is to use cell permeable low-molecular-weight inhibitors specific for the EGFR tyrosine kinase (Levitzki 1990). It has been possible to develop these and phase I trials are starting. Potential problems include toxic effects on normal tissues expressing EGFR. However, there is much redundancy in these pathways in normal tissues and if the tumour has evolved with greater dependence on the EGFR pathway, selectivity should be possible. An example of this in vivo may be the association of high EGFR-expressing tumours with macrophages. As macrophages make EGF, clones with higher EGFR will have a growth advantage and come to dominate the tumour population. They would then be more susceptible to EGFR inhibition because they were selected for predominance of that pathway.

A recent development in antibodies is the ability to generate monoclonal antibodies with much higher affinity than conventional ones, by using sheep to generate the antibodies (Fig. 4). These antibodies are several logs higher in affinity and may have advantages for prodrug targeting by persisting longer and loading more at the target site. Similarly, scfv versions may have better penetration and longer tissue residence. A direct comparison is needed with conventional antibodies to the same targets.

5.7 Conclusions

Since the EGFR was cloned and its role as an oncogene demonstrated, there has been a large amount of clinical evidence to show it is a rational target for selective antitumour therapy. Advances in antibody technology and high output screening have generated a range of drugs against the EGFR, which are now in phase I trial. It will be important to conduct these trials in ways that may differ from conventional phase II trials. Thus, the EGFR level in the tumours should be known, and endpoint might be stabilisation of tumour growth or alterations in metabolism monitored by positron emission tomography scan rather than regression if the drugs are used as single agents. Finally, these approaches are much more likely to be effective when used in the adjuvant situation against small micrometastases, in combination with chemotherapy.

Acknowledgements. The work of the authors' laboratory is supported by the Imperial Cancer Research Fund. Thanks also to Mrs. Elizabeth Clemson for preparing and typing the manuscript.

References

Cuarteroplaza A, Martinezmiralles E, Rosell R, Vadellnadal C, Farre M, Real FX (1996a) Radiolocalization of squamous lung-carcinoma with i-131-labeled epidermal growth-factor. Clin Cancer Res 2:13–20
Earp HS, Dawson TL, Li X, Yu H (1995) Heterodimerization and functional interaction between EGF receptor family members – a new signaling paradigm with implications for breast-cancer research. Breast Cancer Res Treat 35:115–132
Fitzgerald D, Pastan I (1989) Targeted toxin therapy for the treatment of cancer. J Natl Cancer Inst 81:1455–1463

Fox SB, Leek RD, Smith K, Hollyer J, Greenall M, Harris AL (1994a) Tumour angiogenesis in node-negative breast carcinomas – relationship with epidermal growth factor receptor, oestrogen receptor and survival. Br Cancer Treat Rev 29:109116

Fox SB, Smith K, Hollyer J, Greenall M, Hastrich D, Harris AL (1994b) The epidermal growth factor receptor as a prognostic marker: results of 370 patients and review of 3009 patients. Br J Cancer 29:41–49

Goldstein NI, Prewett M, Zuklys K, Rockwell P, Mendelsohn J (1995) Biological efficacy of a chimeric antibody to the epidermal growth-factor receptor in a human tumor xenograft model. Clin Cancer Res 1:1311–1318

Groenen LC, Nice EC, Burgess AW (1994) Structure-function-relationships for the EGF/tgf-alpha family of mitogens. Growth Factors 11:235–257

Harris AL (1990) Commentary: the epidermal growth factor receptor as a target for therapy. Cancer Cells 2:321–323

Harris AL (1991) Growth factors and receptors in cancer. Curr Opin Biotechnol 2:260–268

Horak E, Leek R, Klenk N, LeJeune S, Smith K, Stuart N, Greenall M, Stepniewska K, Harris AL (1992) Angiogenesis, assessed by platelet/endothelial cell adhesion molecule antibodies, as an indicator of node metastasis and survival in breast cancer. Lancet 340:1120–1124

Kirk J, Carmichael J, Stratford IJ, Harris AJ (1994) Selective toxicity of TGF-α-PE40 to ERFR-positive cell lines: selection protection of low EGFR-expressing cell lines by EGF. Br J Cancer 69:988–994

Klijn JC, Berns PM, Schmitz PI, Foekens JA (1992) The clinical significance of epidermal growth factor receptor (EGF-R) in human breast cancer: a review on 5232 patients. Endocr Rev 13:3–17

Kroning R, Jones JA, Horn DK, Chuang CC, Sanga R, Los G, Howell SB, Christen RD (1995) Enhancement of drug-sensitivity of human malignancies by epidermal growth-factor. Br J Cancer 72:615–619

Leek RD, Kaklarvianis L, Pezzella F, Gatter KC, Harris AL (1994) BCL-2 in normal human breast and carcinoma, association with oestrogen receptor positive, epidermal growth factor receptor negative tumours and in situ cancer. Br J Cancer 69:135–139

Lejeune S, Leek R, Horak E, Plowman C, Greenall M, Harris AL (1993) Amphiregulin, epidermal growth factor receptor and oestrogen receptor expression in human primary breast cancer. Cancer Res 53:3597–3602

Levitzki A (1990) Tyrphostins – potential antiproliferative agents and novel molecular tools. Biochem Pharmacol 40:913–918

Lupu R, Cardillo M, Harris L, Hijazi M, Rosenberg K (1995) Interaction between erbb- receptors and heregulin in breast-cancer tumor progression and drugresistance. Semin Cancer Biol 6:135–145

Neal DE, Marsh C, Bennett MK, Abel PD, Sainsbury JRC, Hall RR, Harris AL
(1985) Epidermal growth factor receptors in human bladder cancer: comparison of invasive and superficial tumours. Lancet I:366–368

Neal DE, Sharples L, Smith K, Fennelly J, Hall RR, Harris AL (1990) The epidermal growth factor receptor and the prognosis of bladder cancer. Cancer
65:1619–1625

Newby JC, Ahern RP, Leek RD, Smith IE, Harris AL, Dowsett M (1995) Immunohistochemical assay for epidermal growth-factor receptor on paraf-
finembedded sections – validation against ligand-binding assay and clinical
relevance in breast-cancer. Br J Cancer 71:1237–1242

Nicholson S, Halcrow P, Sainsbury JRC, Angus B, Chambers P, Farndon JR,
Harris AL (1988) Epidermal growth factor receptor status associated with
failure of primary endocrine therapy in elderly postmenopausal patients
with breast cancer. Br J Cancer 58:810–814

Nicholson S, Sainsbury JRC, Halcrow P, Chambers P, Farndon JR, Harris AL
(1989) Epidermal growth factor receptor expression is associated with lack
of response to endocrine therapy in patients with recurrent breast cancer.
Lancet I:182–185

Normanno N, Kim N, Wen DZ, Smith K, Harris AL, Plowman G, Colletta G,
Ciardiello F, Salomon DS (1995) Expression of messenger-RNA for amphiregulin, heregulin and cripto-1 3 new members of the epidermal growth factor family, in human breast carcinomas. Breast Cancer Res Treat 35:293–297

O'Sullivan C, Lewis CE, Harris AL, McGee J0 (1993) Secretion of epidermal
growth factor by macrophages associated with breast carcinoma. Lancet
342:148–149

Patterson AV, Zhang H, Moghaddam A, Bicknell R, Talbot DC, Stratford IJ,
Harris AL (1995) Increased sensitivity to the prodrug 5'-deoxy-5-
fluorouridine and modulation of 5-fluoro-2'-deozyuridine sensitivity in
MCF-7 cells transfected with thymidine phosphorylase. Br J Cancer
72:669–675

Petrangeli E, Lubrano C, Ravenna L, Vacca A, Cardillo MR, Salvatori L,
Sciarra F, Frati L, Gulino A (1995) Gene methylation of estrogen and epidermal growth factor receptors in neoplastic and perineopiastic breast tissues. Br J Cancer 72:973–975

Rao RK, Shantaram M, Aroor AR, Raja A, Davis TP, Rao A (1996) Molecular
variants of epidermal growth-factor in malignant astrocytoma. Peptides
17:179–181

Saeki T, Salomon DS, Johnson GR, Gullick WJ, Mandal K, Yamagami K,
Moriwaki S, Tanada M, Takashima S, Tahara E (1995) Association of epidermal growth factor-related peptides and type-1 receptor tyrosine kinase
receptors with prognosis of human colorectal carcinomas. Jpn J Clin Oncol
25:240–249

Scher HI, Sarkis A, Reuter V, Cohen D, Netto G, Petrylak D, Lianes P, Fuks Z, Mendelsohn J, Cordoncardo C (1995) Changing pattern of expression of the epidermal growth-factor receptor and transforming growth-factor-alpha in the progression of prostatic neoplasms. Clin Cancer Res 1:545–550

Schober R, Bilzer T, Waha A, Reifenberger G, Wechsler W, Vondeimling A, Wiestler OD, Westphal M, Kemshead JT, Vega F (1995) The epidermal growth-factor receptor in glioblastoma – genomic amplification, protein expression, and patient survival-data in a therapeutic trial. Clin Neuropathol 14:169–174

Tosi E, Valota O, Negri DRM, Adobati E, Mazzoni A, Meazza R, Ferrini S, Colnaghi MI, Canevari S (1995) Antitumor efficacy of an anti-epidermal-growth-factor receptor monoclonal-antibody and its f(ab')(2) fragment against high-EGFR-expressing and low-EGFR-expressing carcinomas in nude-mice. Int J Cancer 62:643–650

Toyoda H, Komurasaki T, Uchida D, Takayama Y, Isobe T, Okuyama T, Hanada K (1995) Epiregulin – a novel epidermal growth-factor with mitogenic activity for rat primary hepatocytes. J Biol Chem 270:7495–7500

van Agthoven T, Timmermans M, Dorssers LCJ, Henzen-Logmans SC (1995) Expression of oestrogen, progesterone and epidermal growth factor receptors in primary and metastatic breast cancer. Int J Cancer 63:790–793

Veale D, Kerr N, Gibson GJ, Harris AL (1989) Characterisation of epidermal growth factor receptors in primary non-small cell lung cancer. Cancer Res 49:1313–1317

Veale D, Kerr N, Gibson GJ, Kelly PJ, Harris AL (1993) The relationship of quantitative epidermal growth factor receptor expression in non-small cell lung cancer to long term survival. Br J Cancer 68:162–165

Wikstrand CJ, Hale LP, Batra SK, Hill ML, Humphrey PA, Kurpad SN, McLendon RE, Moscatello D, Pegram CN, Reist CJ (1995) Monoclonal antibodies against EGFRviii are tumor-specific and react with breast and lung carcinomas and malignant gliomas. Cancer Res 55:3140–3148

Wright C, Angus B, Nicholson S, Sainsbury JRC. Cairns J, Gullick WJ, Kelly P, Harris AL, Horne CHW (1989) Expression of c-erbB-2 oncoprotein: a prognostic indicator in breast cancer. Cancer Res 49:2087–2090

Wright C, Cairns J, Cantwell BJ, Cattan AR, Hall AG, Harris AL, Horne CHW (1992a) Response to mitoxantrone in advanced breast cancer: correlation with expression of c-erbB-2 protein and glutathione S-transferases. Br J Cancer 65:271–274

Wright C, Nicholson S, Angus B, Sainsbury JRC, Farndon J, Cairns J, Harris AL, Horne CHW (1992b) Relationship between c-erbB-2 protein product expression and response to endocrine therapy in advanced breast cancer. Br J Cancer 65:118–121

6 erbB Signalling and Endocrine Sensitivity of Human Breast Cancer

R.I. Nicholson, J.M.W. Gee, H. Jones, M.E. Harper,
A.E. Wakeling, P. Willsher and J.F.R. Robertson

6.1 Introduction

The development and progression of cancer is believed to involve multiple genetic events occurring in those pathways which regulate the fundamental processes of cellular survival, proliferation and differentiation. Such changes, which are likely to occur through both oncogenic activation and via the loss of suppressor gene function (Walker and Varley 1993), ultimately alter the phenotype of cancer cells and allow them to thrive under conditions in which their normal counterparts remain severely growth restrained (Gee et al. 1996; Nicholson and Gee 1996).

A common (and perhaps even inevitable) consequence of such changes in breast neoplasia is the apparent loss of cellular sensitivity to

an important class of growth-promoting molecules, the steroid hormones, a feature perhaps coupled with an increased reliance on growth
factor-mediated pathways (Gee et al. 1996; Nicholson and Gee 1996).
Endocrine insensitivity is manifested clinically either by an initial failure to respond to antihormonal measures (e.g. antioestrogens, aromatase
inhibitors, luteinizing hormone-releasing hormone, LH-RH, agonists
and progestins; reviewed in Nicholson et al. 1986, 1992, 1993a; Nicholson 1993) or, if a primary tumour remission does occur, through the
subsequent progressive acquisition of endocrine resistance (Patterson
1981).

An on-going focus of the research activity performed within the
Tenovus Cancer Research Centre is the precise delineation of those
aspects of the breast cancer phenotype which are responsible for (rather
than merely associated with) primary and acquired endocrine resistance.
In this light, the current article explores the evidence linking one such
phenotypic parameter, elevated expression of the epidermal growth factor receptor (EGFR) and/or additional members of the erbB membrane-
spanning tyrosine kinase receptor family, with loss of endocrine response and growth control. It is obvious that such studies are an
essential prerequisite to the rational use of EGFR-selective tyrosine
kinase inhibitors (Wakeling et al. 1994, 1996) and other innovative
anti-growth factor regimes (Gee et al. 1996; Nicholson and Gee 1996;
Ennis et al. 1991; Levitzki 1994; Staebler et al. 1994) in the control of
endocrine insensitive and resistant breast cancer growth.

6.2 Cellular Levels and Distribution of the EGFR Protein

More than a decade has now elapsed since the first report describing the
presence of EGFR in some human breast tumours (Sainsbury et al.
1985). Of particular interest was the observation that prominence of the
protein was associated with a significantly worsened patient prognosis
(Sainsbury et al. 1985; Hainsworth et al. 1991; Klijn et al. 1992).

The principal method of detection employed in these early studies
was the ligand-binding assay, revealing a 40% EGFR positivity rate
(Sainsbury et al. 1985; Hainsworth et al. 1991; Klijn et al. 1992).
However, subsequent methodological development has provided immunocytochemical procedures of markedly superior sensitivity to their

biochemical predecessors. These new technologies are equally applicable to frozen material (Nicholson et al. 1993b, 1994b; McClelland et al. 1994) and, after antigen retrieval, to routinely-fixed, paraffin-embedded tissues (Newby et al. 1995). Our own studies (Nicholson et al. 1993b, 1994b; McClelland et al. 1994) have strongly-favoured immunocytochemistry, since this technique not only has the unique ability of localizing the EGFR protein to its cellular origin, but furthermore enables direct comparison to be made with the expression of other relevant immunohistochemically detected biological endpoints. These include receptor ligands (e.g. transforming growth factor-α, TGF-α; Nicholson et al. 1994a), components of the signal transduction pathway subsequently employed on receptor activation (e.g. the nuclear transcription factors Fos and Myc; Gee et al. 1995a), and other erbB family members (e.g. c-erbB-2 protein; Nicholson et al. 1993).

A universal observation from studies employing either ligand-binding assays or immunohistochemistry is that expression of the EGFR protein is highly variable within the breast cancer population (Fig. 1a), ranging from essentially EGFR negativity through to high levels of positivity (Nicholson et al. 1993b, 1994b; McClelland et al. 1994). In this light, detailed evaluation of our own series revealed total EGFR immunostaining to consist of cytoplasmic immunoreactivity, a continuous variable present in the majority of primary and locally advanced breast cancers (Fig. 1a), with EGFR membrane staining also being detectable in 50% of cases (Nicholson et al. 1993b, 1994b; McClelland et al. 1994). In comparison, normal breast epithelia (Walker et al. 1991) and hormone-sensitive MCF-7 human breast cancer cells (Gee and Nicholson, unpublished data) can be shown to contain only very weak cytoplasmic immunostaining. We have observed that the majority of EGFR membrane positive tumour specimens are poorly differentiated grade III cancers (Fig. 1a) frequently lacking tubular differentiation, with inherently high levels of nuclear pleomorphism and mitotic activity. In contrast, however, the remaining predominantly EGFR membrane negative tumours comprise more well-differentiated cancer types (grade I and II tumours; $\chi^2=8.91$, $p<0.002$), phenotypically reminiscent of the normal breast epithelium (Walker et al. 1991).

Subsequent subdivision of this data by the oestrogen receptor (ER) status of the tumours (Nicholson et al. 1993b, 1994b; McClelland et al. 1994) dramatically demonstrates that EGFR membrane immunostain-

EGFR HScore

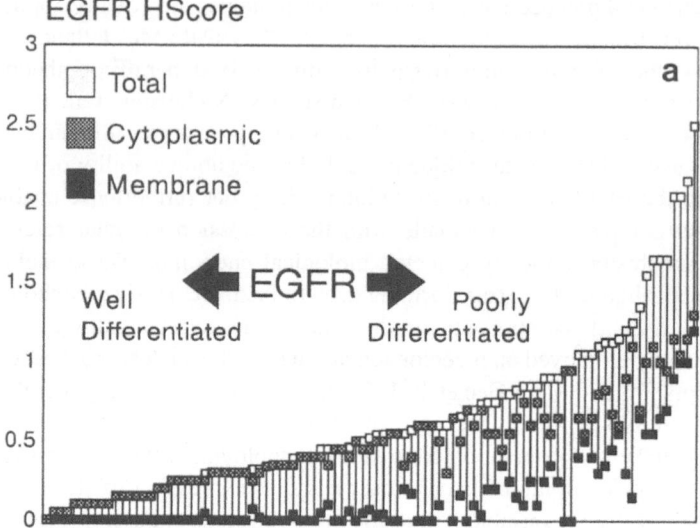

EGFR HScore

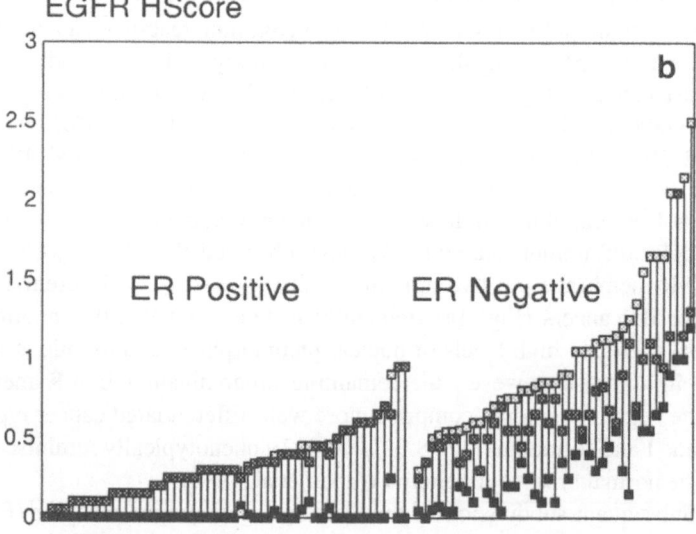

Fig. 1. Legend see p. 109

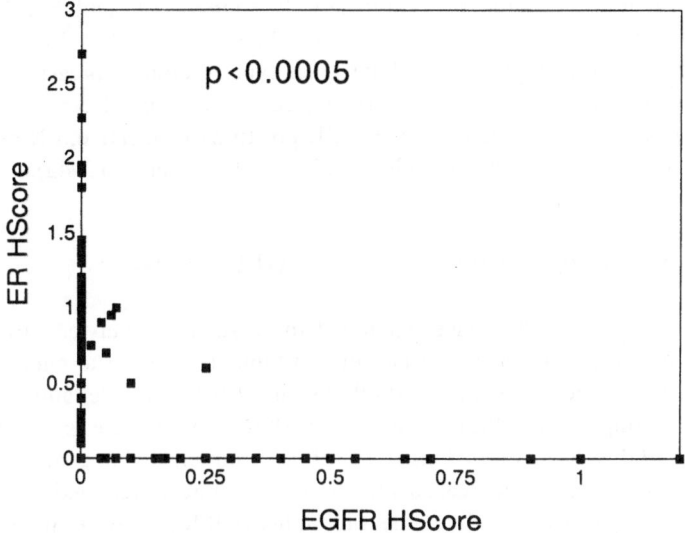

Fig. 2. Inverse association between nuclear oestrogen receptor and epidermal growth factor receptor membrane immunostaining

ing is almost entirely confined to ER-negative disease (Fig. 1b), generating the commonly noted inverse association between these two parameters (Fig. 2; also reviewed in Klijn et al. 1992). Indeed, on the few occasions when we have observed EGFR membrane-positive cells within ER-positive cancers, these cells normally comprise merely a minority phenotype, with co-expression of EGFR membrane and nuclear ER immunostaining within individual tumour cells being conspicuously absent. It is certainly likely that ER and membrane-associated EGFRs are mutually exclusive within tumour cells, as evidenced by our observation that dual immunohistochemical assays, which are

◀ **Fig. 1a,b.** Distribution of the epidermal growth factor receptor (*EGFR*) in clinical breast cancer specimens before (**a**) and after (**b**) subdivision according to oestrogen receptor (*ER*) status. EGFR and ER immunocytochemical assays and HScore staining assessments were performed as described previously (Nicholson et al. 1993b, 1994b; McClelland et al. 1994)

known to be capable of simultaneously staining ER and EGFR in ER-positive human breast cancer cells (Sharma et al. 1994b), fail to reveal the double-positive cellular phenotype in clinical breast cancer specimens (Sharma et al. 1994a). Indeed, such studies have revealed only three cellular phenotypes, i.e. ER-positive/ER-negative, ER-negative/EGFR-positive, and double negativity (Sharma et al. 1994a).

6.3 Endocrine Response and the EGFR Protein

To date, two studies have examined the association between EGFR expression in clinical breast cancer and tumour response to endocrine measures (Nicholson et al. 1989, 1993b, 1994b; McClelland et al. 1994). Importantly, these studies have shown that increases in either total EGFR level or in EGFR membrane immunostaining alone are associated with an increased likelihood of failure to respond to such therapy. This is especially evident in highly EGFR positive tumours, in which elevated receptor levels also appear to correlate with a significantly worsened patient outlook (Nicholson et al. 1993b, 1994b; McClelland et al. 1994), such patients having a median time to death of only 12 months in advanced disease (Nicholson et al. 1993).

Subdivision of our EGFR immunocytochemical data according to ER status clearly demonstrates that the response rate to endocrine measures is extremely low in women with EGFR-positive/ER-negative disease (Nicholson et al. 1993b, 1994b; McClelland et al. 1994), in agreement the results of S. Nicholson et al. (1989). Indeed, in our own study, only 1/40 such patients appeared to benefit from endocrine treatment, with this tumour phenotype also being associated with extremely poor survival characteristics. In contrast, approximately 60% (28/45) of women with ER-positive disease showed some degree of response, with 33% (15/45) obtaining complete or partial remissions (Nicholson et al. 1993b, 1994b; McClelland et al. 1994). Interestingly, however, the presence of EGFR membrane immunostaining within ER-positive cancers does not necessarily preclude an initial response to endocrine therapy (Nicholson et al. 1993b, 1994b; McClelland et al. 1994).

The above data raise several important points worthy of further discussion regarding the role (if any) played by the epidermal growth factor receptor in directing endocrine response in breast cancer:

1. Since ER-negative cancers by definition lack the cellular machinery necessary to directly respond to anti-oestrogens (Nicholson 1992), is the EGFR protein associated with such tumours merely a minor constituent of the endocrine unresponsive phenotype or is it (perhaps together with further elements of the erbB signalling pathway) a fundamental component of the growth control mechanism in ER-negative cells?

2. Since remissions seen in ER-positive tumours occur despite their cellular EGFR content, it appears that EGFR expression is unlikely to be of major significance in determining initial (primary) endocrine resistance observed in ER-positive disease. However, is it possible that acquired endocrine resistance ultimately demonstrated by many patients with ER-positive disease may have its origins in the EGFR/erbB signalling pathway, notably in the selective outgrowth of any population of endocrine unresponsive EGFR-positive/ER-negative cells?

6.3.1 Does EGFR (and c-erbB-2 Protein) Signalling Play an Important Role in the Growth Control of ER-Negative Disease?

A convenient means of assessing the growth characteristics of breast cancer has involved immunostaining frozen (Nicholson et al. 1993; Bouzubar et al. 1989; Locker et al. 1992) or, more recently, paraffin-embedded (Gee et al. 1995a) tissue sections with Ki-67 antibodies which can detect a proliferation-associated antigen (Gerdes et al. 1983). Using this methodology, the observed proliferative index, in common with EGFR immunostaining, is revealed to be highly variable in breast cancer, furthermore relating closely to patient prognosis. In this light, increasing levels of Ki-67 positivity have been shown to correlate with both a shortened disease-free interval and reduced survival (Bouzubar et al. 1989; Locker et al. 1992). Interestingly, an elevated Ki-67 score is also associated with an increased likelihood of failure to respond to endocrine therapy (Nicholson et al. 1991, 1993).

In order to address the question as to whether the EGFR is a likely player in the control of ER-negative cell growth, we have completed a detailed examination of the relationship between cellular proliferation, as assessed by such Ki-67 immunostaining, and the level of EGFR

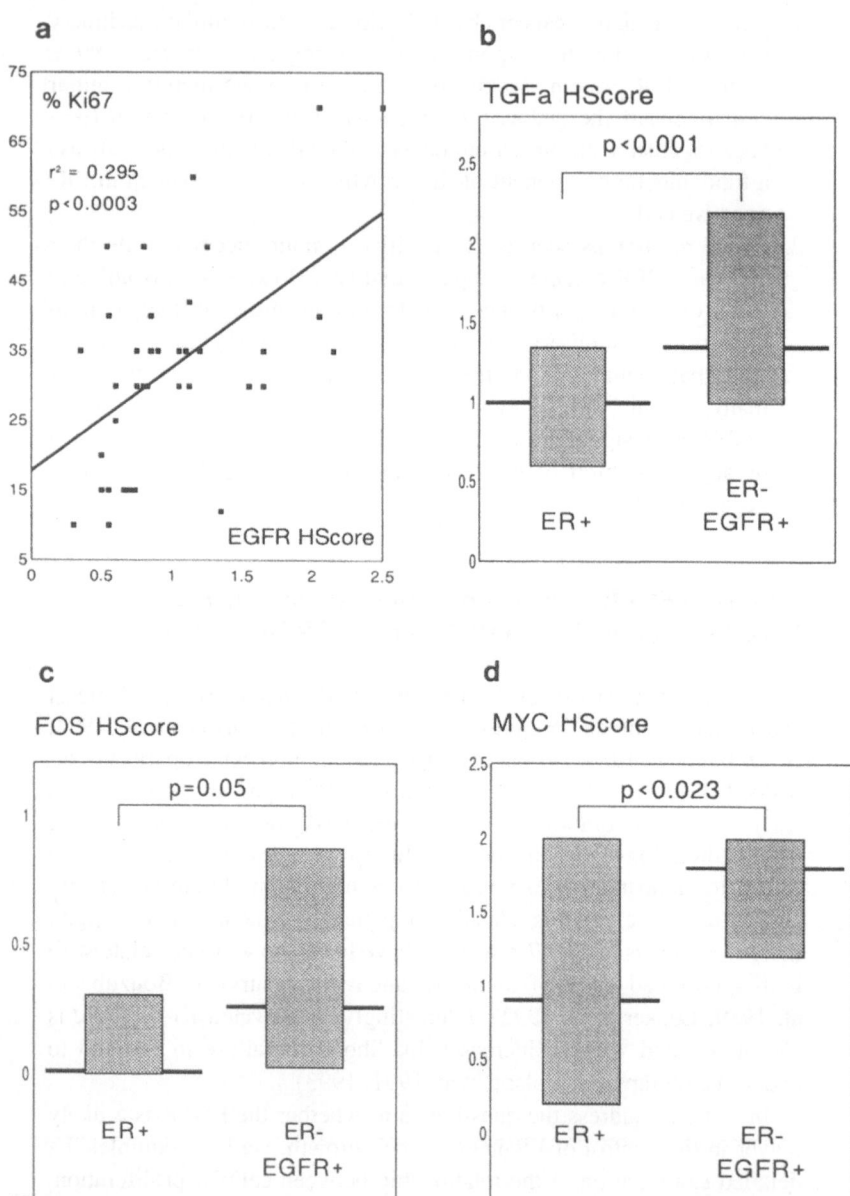

Fig. 3. Legend see p. 113

positivity in serial sections of steroid receptor-negative breast cancers (Nicholson et al. 1993b, 1994a; Gee et al. 1995b; Bouzubar et al. 1989). As may be seen in Fig. 3a, a highly significant positive correlation can be demonstrated between these two parameters, with the proportion of Ki-67 positive tumour cells increasing in parallel with escalating total EGFR levels. This association is maintained when either membrane or cytoplasmic EGFR immunostaining are examined in isolation (not illustrated).

These results certainly imply an integral role for the EGFR in directing the growth of ER-negative cells, a hypothesis further strengthened by our observation that many additional key elements of the EGFR growth signalling pathway are also conspicuous in such clinical samples. Thus, all tumours express immunodetectable levels of TGF-α (Nicholson et al. 1994a), a potent mitogen for breast cancer cells in vitro (Bates et al. 1988), with the cellular concentration of this important EGFR ligand being notably higher in EGFR-positive/ER-negative tumours than in ER-positive disease (Fig. 3b). Equally, EGFR-positive/ER-negative tumours also demonstrate increased levels of the nuclear transcription factors Fos (Gee et al. 1995b; Fig. 3c) and Myc (Nicholson and Gee, unpublished data, Fig 3d), proteins which are believed to comprise an important part of growth factor-driven growth responses in vitro (Landes and Spelsberg 1992).

However, the correlation between EGFR and Ki-67 immunostaining appears to be dramatically perturbed by the presence of an additional erbB family member (Prigent and Lemoine 1992), the c-erbB-2 gene product, a transmembrane receptor overexpressed in 40% of ER-negative breast tumours (Nicholson et al. 1990, 1993; Slamon et al. 1987). Thus, while the proportion of Ki-67 positive tumour cells increases in parallel with increasing EGFR immunostaining in c-erbB-2 negative disease (Fig. 4a), this relationship is notably lacking in ER-negative/c-erbB-2 positive breast cancers (Fig. 4b). Although the precise molecular

---

◄ **Fig. 3a–d.** Characteristics of oestrogen receptor (*ER*)-negative tumours disease. Epidermal growth factor receptor (*EGFR*) and Ki-67 (**a**), transforming growth factor-α (*TGF-α*; **b**), Fos (**c**), and Myc expression (**d**). All immunocytochemical assays and HScore staining assessments were performed as described previously (Nicholson et al. 1993b, 1994a; Gee et al. 1995b; Bouzubar et al. 1989)

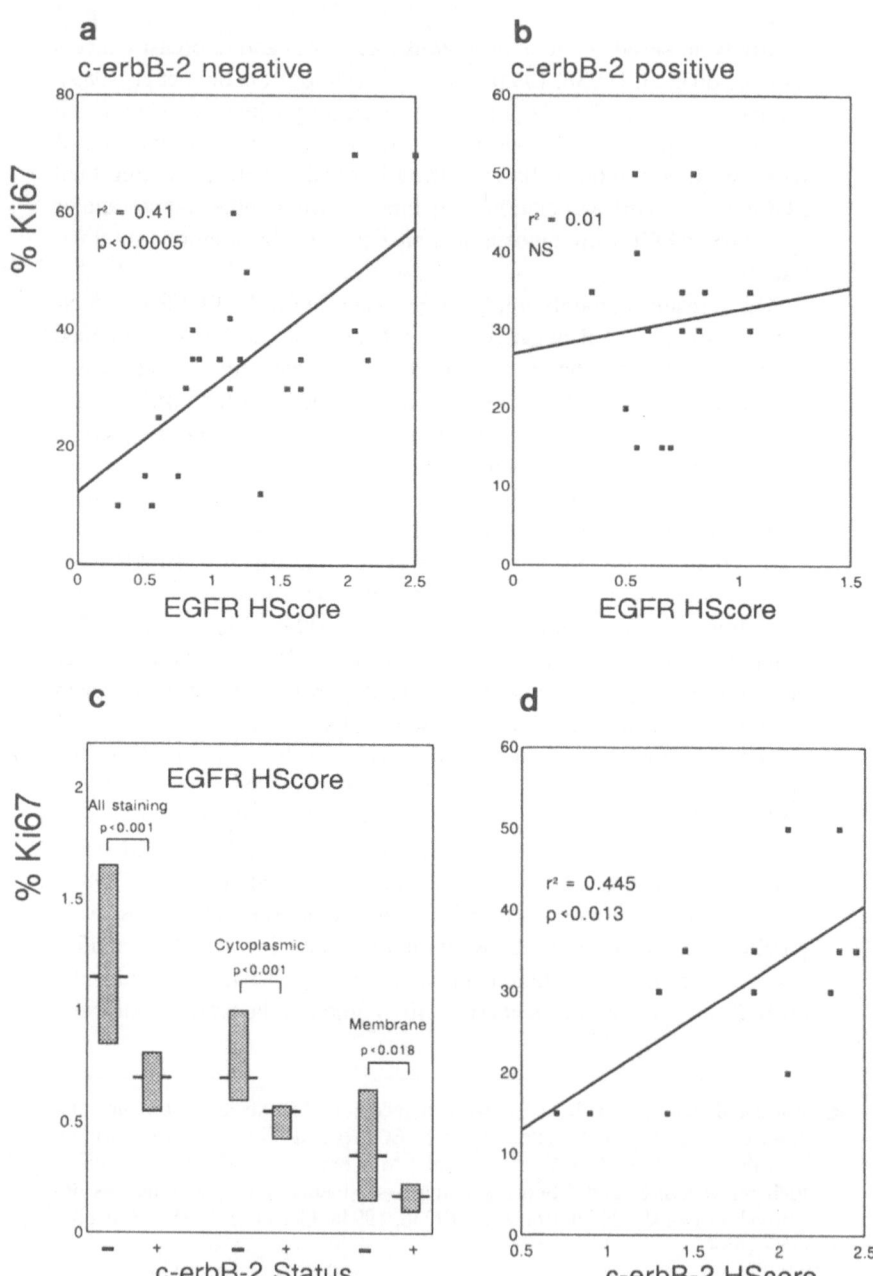

Fig. 4. Legend see p. 115

mechanisms underlying this distortion are currently unknown, it is interesting that EGFR levels are observed to be significantly diminished in such c-erbB-2 positive breast cancers (Fig. 4c), a feature perhaps allowing an "uncoupling" of any influence the EGFR may have on cellular proliferation. Furthermore, c-erbB-2 protein levels are highly variable in ER-negative/c-erbB-2-positive disease (Nicholson et al. 1993) and are directly related to those seen for Ki-67 (Fig. 4d). Amplification of the c-erbB-2 gene (Slamon et al. 1987) and the resultant overexpression of its protein product (Nicholson et al. 1993) appears, therefore, not only to be able to circumvent the functional activity of the EGFR in ER-negative disease, but importantly may provide an alternative stimulus for constituent cell growth.

These above data, although not constituting definitive proof that cellular levels of the EGFR and c-erbB-2 proteins are directly responsible for the prevailing proliferation rate in ER-negative disease, certainly provide some encouragement that new anti-growth factor regimes (Wakeling et al. 1994, 1996; Ennis et al. 1991; Levitzki 1994; Staebler et al. 1994) directed towards key members of the erbB receptor family (Prigent and Lemoine 1992) may be of genuine therapeutic benefit in ER-negative, endocrine-insensitive breast cancer. This concept is, in part, supported by recent preclinical in vitro studies examining the effects of EGFR-selective tyrosine kinase inhibitors [e.g. 4(3-chloroanilinoquinazoline), CAQ; Wakeling et al. 1994, 1996] on steroid hormone receptor-negative cancer cell lines. Encouragingly, these compounds can be demonstrated to specifically block the growth promoting effects of EGFR ligands (i.e. TGF-α and EGF; Jones et al. 1996a) applied exogenously to such cultures (Jones et al. 1996b). Indeed, in a number of instances, the tyrosine kinase inhibitors are also effective in reducing cell basal growth under serum-free conditions (Jones et al. 1996b). Fortuitously, therefore, while it appears that many such cells are certainly capable of synthesizing and secreting ligands which can acti-

---

◀ **Fig. 4a–d.** Influence of the c-erbB-2 protein on the biology of oestrogen receptor-negative breast cancer, notably on the relationship between epidermal growth factor receptor (EGFR) and Ki-67 expression (**a, b**) and EGFR immunostaining (**c**). **d** Relationship between c-erbB-2 expression and Ki-67. The c-erbB-2 immunocytochemical assay was performed as described previously (Nicholson et al. 1993b)

Cell number (10⁻³)

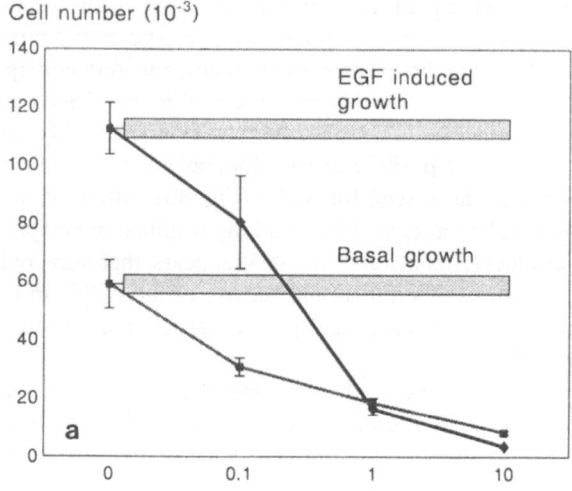

Cell number (X10⁻³)

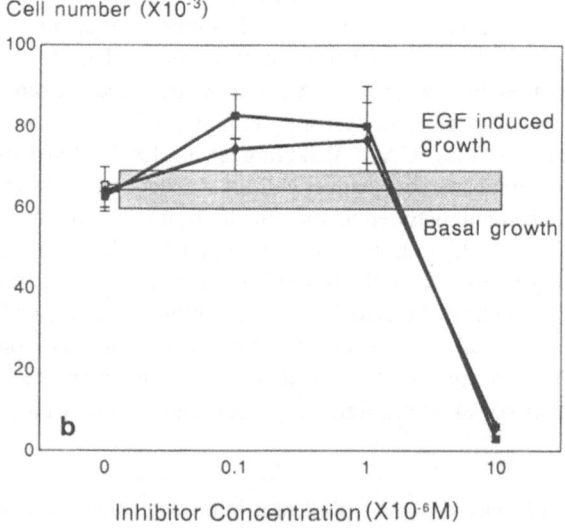

Inhibitor Concentration (X10⁻⁶M)

Fig. 5. Legend see p. 117

vate the EGFR in an autocrine manner, it is nevertheless likely that such pathways may be equally susceptible to the inhibitory properties of these new compounds. This feature is exemplified by our studies (Jones et al. 1996a,b) examining the DU145 human prostate cancer cell line (Mickey et al. 1980), shown in Fig. 5a. These cells are androgen receptor (AR) negative, expressing high EGFR levels on their cell membranes and, perhaps predictably, demonstrating increased growth on exogenous application of EGF (Jones et al. 1996a,b; Eaton et al. 1990). They also synthesize and secrete the EGFR ligand TGF-α in culture, but retain sensitivity to growth inhibition by tyrosine kinase inhibitors at physiological concentrations which are known to target exogenous EGF-promoted growth (Jones et al. 1996a,b). Interestingly, however, contrasting results have been obtained using a similarly AR-negative prostate cancer cell line, PC3 (Kaighn et al. 1979). Such cells are again EGFR positive (Eaton et al. 1996); however, their EGFR immunostaining is exclusively cytoplasmic (Harper and Nicholson, unpublished data), while their basal growth is resistant both to stimulation by exogenously applied EGF and to inhibition by tyrosine kinase inhibitors until nonphysiological concentrations of the drug are employed (Fig. 5b). Such results certainly point to a diminished importance of the EGFR-directed mitogenic pathway in these cells, and we believe that an alternative stimulus for PC3 cell growth may indeed lie elsewhere, perhaps in their elevated levels of c-erbB-2 immunostaining (Harper and Nicholson, unpublished data).

6.3.2 Does EGFR (and c-erbB-2 Protein) Signalling Play an Important Role in Endocrine Response in ER-Positive Disease?

Our previous studies have shown that median tumour ER levels in ER-positive disease are comparable, irrespective of whether a patient subsequently shows a good primary response to endocrine measures (i.e

---

◀ **Fig. 5a,b.** Effect of the EGFR-selective tyrosine kinase inhibitor 4(3-chloroanilinoquinazoline (CAQ) on the basal and epidermal growth factor (*EGF*)-stimulated growth of DU145 (**a**) and PC3 (**b**) human prostate cancer cells. Cells were grown for 14 days in serum-free DCCM-1 tissue culture medium in the presence or absence of 10 ng/ml EGF and increasing concentrations of CAQ. Cell numbers were assessed in triplicate using a Coulter Counter

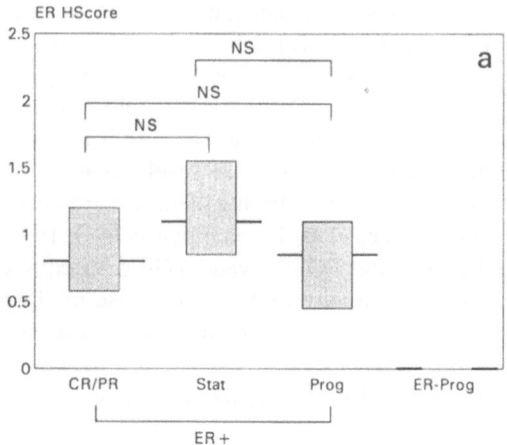

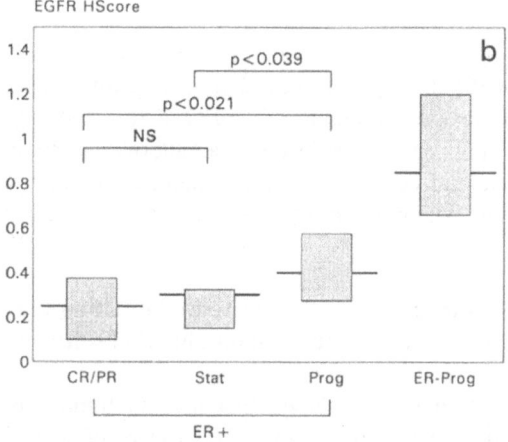

Fig. 6a,b. Relationship between oestrogen receptor (*ER*; **a**) and epidermal growth factor receptor (*EGFR*; **b**) and initial response to endocrine therapy. Patients were assessed for complete or partial responses (CR/PR), static disease (*Stat*, no change) or progression (*Prog*) at 2- to 3-month intervals by UICC criteria (Hayward et al. 1977). As recommended by the British Breast Group, responsive and static disease were only reported after a minimum duration of remission of 6 months (British Breast Group 1974). Tumour samples were assayed immunocytochemically for ER and EGFR as described previously (Nicholson et al. 1993b, 1994b; McClelland et al. 1994)

a complete, CR, or partial, PR, response), has static disease, or in whom disease progresses on such therapy (Fig. 6a). Similarly, although endocrine insensitive, ER-positive tumours do contain slightly higher cytoplasmic EGFR immunostaining than their endocrine responsive counterparts, the levels observed are always markedly reduced over those seen in ER-negative disease, with EGFR membrane staining being notably scarce (Fig. 1b; Fig. 6b). Our studies thus fail to provide evidence for a subpopulation of ER-negative/EGFR membrane-positive cells directing primary endocrine failure within ER-positive disease.

In a recent review of both the clinical and experimental data in breast cancer it has been proposed (Robertson 1996) that the ER-positive phenotype is relatively stable, with true ER negativity being rarely emergent during endocrine manipulation. Initial suggestion of the stability of ER in endocrine-treated breast tumours was to be found in a previous study (Robertson et al. 1991) in which sequential biopsies from patients receiving tamoxifen reported that ER continued to be expressed after 1–4 months of therapy. At the point of these repeat biopsies none of the tumours had developed acquired resistance and therefore it was assumed that it was too early to identify any change in ER phenotype. More recently we have observed that few initially ER-positive tumours are classifiable as ER-negative at the time of acquisition of endocrine resistance and patient relapse (Nicholson and Robertson, unpublished data). There is similarly no evidence to suggest that a parallel accrual of EGFR membrane immunostaining, which would perhaps mark an outgrowth of ER-negative/EGFR-positive cells, occurs in such tumours (Nicholson and Robertson, unpublished data).

While acquisition of the ER-negative phenotype is thus obviously extremely rare (Robertson 1996), we have also recently observed that a fall in tumour ER level appears to be almost universal in patients undergoing tamoxifen treatment. However, this decrease fails to preclude responses, which are still obvious in many patients at 6 months. Furthermore, such anti-oestrogen-induced decreases in ER appear independent of any concurrent alterations in EGFR levels (Nicholson and Robertson, unpublished data).

These results therefore indicate that it is highly unlikely that either primary or acquired endocrine resistance is commonly resultant from any significant outgrowth of endocrine unresponsive ER-negative/EGFR membrane-positive cell phenotype under the selective pres-

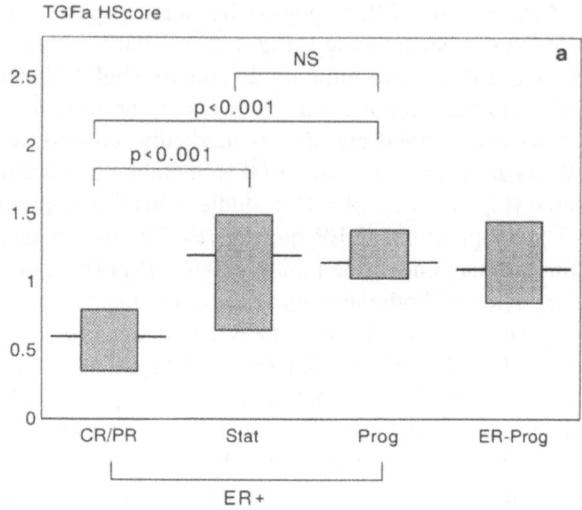

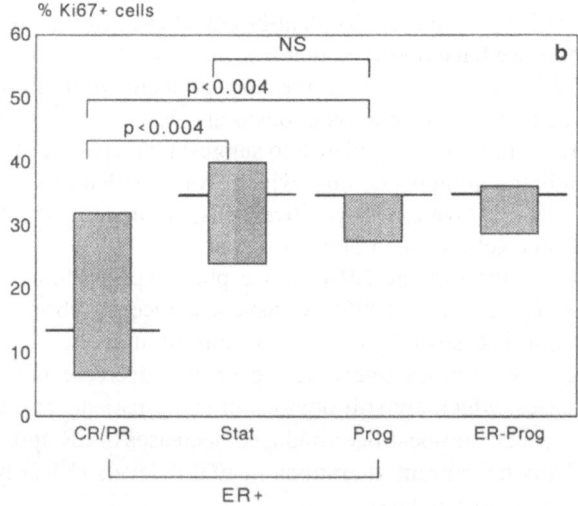

Fig. 7. Legend see p. 121

sure of an altered steroid hormone environment. However, we do have limited evidence implicating further components of the erbB signalling pathway in the perturbation of endocrine responsiveness within steroid receptor-positive disease.

In this light, we have identified that elevated expression of the EGFR ligand TGF-α is associated with a failure of ER-positive breast tumours to respond in vivo to endocrine therapy (Nicholson et al. 1994a), with higher levels of this growth factor being largely confined to either static or progressive disease (Fig. 7a). Our clinical studies also indicate that expression of the nuclear transcription factors Fos and Myc, potentially important players in TGF-α-driven mitogenic responses in vitro, may similarly be elevated in endocrine unresponsive ER-positive tumours in vivo (Gee et al. 1995b). Despite such tumours generally also having an elevated proliferative status (Fig. 7b; Nicholson et al. 1994a; Gee et al. 1995b), however, significant correlations between individual TGF-α/Fos/Myc and Ki-67 immunostaining values are nevertheless notably lacking (Nicholson et al. 1994a; Gee et al. 1995b). Indeed, elevated TGF-α levels (Gee et al. 1996; Nicholson et al. 1995a) have been reported to parallel decreases in Ki-67 levels (Clarke et al. 1993) following short-term exposure to tamoxifen (Dowsett, personal communication), although this is certainly controversial (Noguchi et al. 1993), while overexpression of an additional EGFR ligand (EGF) that occurs subsequent to EGF gene transfer into T-47D breast cancer cells is reported to diminish the growth inhibitory effects of both anti-oestrogens and progestins by mechanisms which are independent of the prevailing cell proliferation rate (Murphy and Dotzlaw 1989). Such data infer that EGFR ligands such as TGF-α do not play an integral role in directly orchestrating the mitogenic process within ER-positive tumours. However, an indirect role for TGF-α may still be feasible, with tumour-secreted TGF-α perhaps driving noncancerous elements within tumours in a paracrine manner to subsequently diminish the endocrine responsiveness of neighbouring tumour epithelial cells. It is also possible that increased TGF-α expression may merely comprise part of the

◀ **Fig. 7.** Relationship between TGF-α (**a**) and Ki-67 (**b**) immunostaining and initial response to endocrine therapy. Response details are as described in Fig. 6 and assay details are as in Fig. 3

endocrine insensitive phenotype, where it could be important in additional aspects of tumour biology (Gee et al. 1996; Nicholson and Gee 1996). In this light, there is evidence implicating the growth factor in angiogenesis (Okumura et al. 1992), while both TGF-α and EGF appear able to inhibit the spontaneous onset of apoptotic DNA cleavage seen in ovarian granules cell cultures (an effect that is counteracted by tyrosine kinase inhibitors; Tilly et al. 1992).

Further supportive evidence of a diminished role for both TGF-α and EGFR in directing cell proliferation and/or endocrine response in ER-positive disease has arisen from our recent studies examining the growth inhibition effected by the EGFR-selective tyrosine kinase inhibitor CAQ within in vitro models of oestrogen growth-responsive (MCF-7) and -independent (K3) ER-positive breast cancer (Nicholson et al. 1995a,b; Katzenellenbogen et al. 1987). In each instance, and despite K3 cells containing elevated levels of TGF-α (Nicholson et al. 1995a,b; Katzenellenbogen et al. 1987), CAQ was markedly less effective at inhibiting both cell basal and steroid-induced growth (Gee et al. 1996; Nicholson and Gee 1996; Nicholson et al. 1995a,b) in comparison with steroid receptor-negative phenotypes, exemplified by the DU145 cancer cell line (Jones et al. 1996a,b).

Finally, our group has previously failed to demonstrate a convincing relationship between expression of the c-erbB-2 protein and endocrine response in ER-positive disease (Nicholson et al. 1993). Indeed, patient response to endocrine therapy appears to occur irrespective of tumour c-erbB-2 protein status. However, it should be noted that these data sharply contrast with other existing literature, which has demonstrated that the endocrine response rate in ER-positive disease is significantly reduced in the presence of c-erbB-2 positivity (Nicholson et al. 1990). This feature also appears to be associated with the presence of lymph node metastases and reduced patient survival (Nicholson et al. 1990, 1993; Slamon et al. 1987). In all the available data, however, it is apparent that presence of the oncoprotein never totally precludes a response to endocrine therapy, and it is thus evident that additional factors exist which are likely to be more important than c-erbB-2 in determining endocrine response (Gee et al. 1996; Nicholson and Gee 1996).

6.4 Summary

A common phenotypic consequence of the many genetic changes that occur in breast neoplasia is a loss of steroid hormone sensitivity, a feature manifested clinically by primary or acquired resistance to anti-hormones. Increasing evidence suggests this condition may involve an enhanced reliance on growth factor-mediated pathways, notably erbB signalling, and examination of this hypothesis forms the focus of our on-going research.

It appears that the absence of steroid receptor machinery rather than a widespread elevated EGFR expression determines the failure of ER-negative tumours to respond to endocrine therapies. However, we believe that the erbB signalling pathway is far from redundant in these tumours. Our in vivo evidence suggests that both the EGFR and c-erbB-2 proteins are fundamental elements in ER-negative disease growth control, while further erbB pathway components (e.g. TGF-α, Fos, Myc) are also apparent.

In contrast, neither diminished ER nor elevated EGFR expression appears to be essential in determining any primary endocrine insensitivity demonstrated by ER-positive tumours, although elevated expression of additional erbB pathway components (e.g. TGF-α, Fos, Myc and c-erbB-2 protein) may be important. However, none of these factors appear to direct endocrine unresponsive, ER-positive cell proliferation. Furthermore, it is unlikely that selective outgrowth of endocrine unresponsive, EGFR membrane-positive/ER-negative cells constitutes a major event in ER-positive tumours during their inevitable acquisition of endocrine resistance.

These in vivo data, further supported by in vitro studies, certainly provide encouragement that new anti-growth factor regimes directed towards key members of the erbB receptor family (e.g. tyrosine kinase inhibitors) may be of unique therapeutic benefit in ER-negative, endocrine-insensitive breast cancer. Unfortunately, however, their usefulness in ER-positive disease that exhibits primary or acquired endocrine resistance remains as yet controversial.

124   R.I. Nicholson et al.

References

British Breast Group (1974) Assessment of response to treatment in advanced breast cancer. Lancet 2:38–39

Bates SE, Davidson NE, Valverius EM, Freter CE, Dickson RB, Tam JP, Kudlow JE, Lippman ME, Salomon DS (1988) Expression of transforming growth factor alpha and its messenger ribonucleic acid in human breast cancer: its regulation by estrogen and its possible functional significance. Mol Endocrinol 2:543–555

Bouzubar N, Walker KJ, Griffiths K, Ellis IO, Elston CW, Robertson JFR, Blamey RW, Nicholson RI (1989) Ki-67 immunostaining in primary breast cancer: pathological and clinical associations. Br J Cancer 59:943–947

Clarke RB, Laidlaw IJ, Jones LJ, Howell A, Anderson E (1993) Effect of tamoxifen on Ki-67 labelling index in human breast tumours and its relationship to oestrogen and progesterone receptor status. Br J Cancer 67(3):606–611

Eaton CL, France TD, Harper ME, Davies P (1990) Epidermal growth factor and androgen action in normal and neoplastic cell lines. In: Robel P (ed) Prostate tumours: bulletin of the association for research on tumours of the prostate (artp). ARTP Bull 6:14

Eaton CL, Jones H, Barrow D, Dutkowski C, France TD, Griffiths K (1996) Differential modulation of the effects of epidermal growth factor in prostatic epithelial cell lines by retinoic acid. J Urol (submitted)

Ennis BW, Lippman ME, Dickson RB (1991) The EGF receptor system as a target for antitumour therapy. Cancer Invest 9:553–562

Gee JMW, Douglas-Jones A, Hepburn P, Sharma AK, McClelland RA, Ellis IO, Nicholson RI (1995a) A cautionary note regarding the application of Ki-67 antibodies to paraffin-embedded breast cancers. J Pathol 177:275–284

Gee JMW, Ellis IO, Robertson JFR, Willsher P, McClelland RA, Hewitt KN, Blamey RW, Nicholson RI (1995b) Immunocytochemical localization of FOS protein in human breast cancers and its relationship to a series of prognostic markers and response to endocrine therapy. Int J Cancer 64:269–273

Gee JMW, McClelland RA, Nicholson RI (1996) Growth factors and endocrine sensitivity in breast cancer. In: Pasqualini JR, Katzenellenbogen BS (eds) Molecular and clinical endocrinology. Dekker, New York, pp 169–188

Gerdes J, Schwab U, Lemke H, Stein H (1983) Production of a mouse monoclonal antibody reactive with a human nuclear antigen associated with cell proliferation. Int J Cancer 31:13–20

Hainsworth PJ, Henderson MA, Stillwell RG, Bennett RC (1991) Comparison of EGFR, c-erbB-2 product and ras p21 immunohistochemistry as prognostic markers in primary breast cancer. Eur J Surg Oncol 17:9–15

Hayward JL, Carbonne PP, Heuston JC, Kumaoka S, Rubens R (1977) Assessment of response to therapy in advanced breast cancer. Cancer 39:1289–1293

Jones HE, Eaton CL, Barrow D, Dutkowski CM, Griffiths K (1996a) Comparative studies of the mitogenic effects of epidermal growth factor and transforming growth factor alpha and the expression of various growth factors in neoplastic and non-neoplastic prostatic cell lines. Prostate (in press)

Jones HE, Harper ME, Wakeling AE, Gee JMW, Nicholson RI (1996b) A new EGFR-specific tyosine kinase inhibitor, ZM 252868, reveals a variable growth control mechanism in prostate cancer cell lines. Int J Cancer (submitted)

Kaighn ME, Narayan KS, Ohnuki Y, Lechner JF, Jones LW (1979) Establishment and characterization of a human prostatic carcinoma cell line (PC3). Invest Urol 17(1):16–23

Katzenellenbogen BS, Kendra KL, Norman MJ, Berthois Y (1987) Proliferation, hormone responsiveness and estrogen receptor content of MCF-7 human breast cancer cells grown in short-term and long-term absence of estrogens. Cancer Res 47:4355–4360

Klijn JGM, Berns PM, Schmitz PI, Foekens JA (1992) The clinical significance of epidermal growth factor receptor in human breast cancer: a review on 5232 patients. Endocr Rev 13:3–17

Landers JP, Spelsberg TC (1992) New concepts in steroid hormone action: transcription factors, protooncogenes, and the cascade model for steroid regulation of gene expression. Crit Rev Euk Gene Expr 2:19–63

Levitzki A (1994) Signal-transduction therapy. A novel approach to disease management. Eur J Biochem 226(1):1–13

Locker AP, Birrell K, Bell JA, Nicholson RI, Elston CW, Blamey RW, Ellis IO (1992) Ki-67 immunoreactivity in breast carcinoma: relationships to prognostic variables and short term survival. Eur J Surg Oncol 18:224–229

McClelland RA, Finlay P, Gee JMW, Manning DL, Hoyle H, Ellis IO, Blamey RW, Nicholson RI (1994) Immunocytochemically-localised epidermal growth factor receptor and estrogen receptor in breast cancer: relationship to endocrine therapy. Oncol Life Sci Adv 12:143–155

Mickey DD, Stone KR, Wunderli H, Mickey GH, Paulson DF (1980) Characterization of a human prostate adenocarcinoma cell line (DU145) as a monolayer culture and as a solid tumor in athymic mice. Prog Clin Biol Res 37:67–84

Murphy LC, Dotzlaw H (1989) Endogenous growth factor expression in T-47D human breast cancer cells associated with reduced sensitivity to antiproliferative effects of progestins and antioestrogens. Cancer Res 490:599–604

Newby JC, A'Hern RP, Leek RD, Smith IE, Harris AL, Dowsett M (1995) Immunohistochemical assay for epidermal growth factor receptor on paraffin-embedded sections: validation against ligand-binding assay and clinical relevance in breast cancer. Br J Cancer 71:1237–1242

Nicholson RI (1992) Why ER level may not reflect endocrine responsiveness in breast cancer. Rev Endocr Relat Cancer 40:25–28

Nicholson RI (1993) Recent advances in the antihormonal therapy of breast cancer. Current Opinion in Investigational Drugs. Oncol Endocr Metab 2 (12):1259–1268

Nicholson RI, Gee JMW (1996) Growth factors and endocrine sensitivity in breast cancer. In: Vedeckis W (ed) Hormones and cancer. Birkhauser, Boston, pp 225–260

Nicholson RI, Walker KJ, Davies P (1986) Hormone agonists and antagonists in the treatment of hormone sensitive breast and prostate cancer. Cancer Surv 5:463–486

Nicholson S, Halcrow P, Fardon JR, Sainsbury JRC, Chambers P, Harris AL (1989) Expression of epidermal growth factor receptors associated with lack of response to endocrine therapy in recurrent breast cancer. Lancet i:182–185

Nicholson S, Wright C, Sainsbury JRC, Fardon JR, Harris AL (1990) Epidermal growth factor receptor as a marker of poor prognosis in node-negative breast cancer patients: neu and tamoxifen failure. J Steroid Biochem Mol Biol 37:811–814

Nicholson RI, Bouzubar N, Walker KJ, McClelland RA, Dixon AR, Robertson JFR, Ellis IO, Blamey RW (1991) Hormone sensitivity in breast cancer: influence of heterogeneity of receptor expression and cell proliferation on hormone sensitivity of breast cancer. Eur J Cancer 27:908–913

Nicholson RI, Eaton CL, Manning DL (1992) New developments in the endocrine management of breast cancer. In: Edwards CRW, Lincoln DW (eds) Recent advances in endocrinology and metabolism, vol 4. Churchill Livingstone, New York, pp 150–165

Nicholson RI, Manning DL, Gee JMW (1993a) New antihormonal approaches to breast cancer therapy. Drugs Today 29 (6):363–372

Nicholson RI, McClelland RA, Finlay P, Eaton CL, Gullick WJ, Dixon AR, Robertson JFR, Ellis IO, Blamey RW (1993b) Relationship between EGFR, c-erbB-2 protein expression and Ki-67 immunostaining in breast cancer and hormone sensitivity. Eur J Cancer 29A:1018–1023

Nicholson RI, McClelland RA, Gee JMW, Manning DL, Cannon P, Robertson JFR, Ellis IO, Blamey RW (1994a) Transforming growth factor-α and endocrine sensitivity in breast cancer. Cancer Res 54:1684–1689

Nicholson RI, McClelland RA, Gee JMW, Manning DL, Cannon P, Robertson JFR, Ellis IO, Blamey RW (1994b) Epidermal growth factor receptor expression in breast cancer: association with response to endocrine therapy. Breast Cancer Res Treat 29:117–125

Nicholson RI, Gee JMW, Manning DL, Wakeling AE, Katzenellenbogen BS (1995a) Responses to pure antioestrogens (ICI 164384 and ICI 182780) in oestrogen sensitive and resistant experimental and clinical breast cancer. Ann N Y Acad Sci 761:148–163

Nicholson RI, Gee JMW, Francis AB, Manning DL, Wakeling AE, Katzenellenbogen BS (1995b) Observations arising from the use of pure antioestrogens on oestrogen-responsive (MCF-7) and oestrogen growth-independent (K3) human breast cancer cells. Endocr Relat Cancer 2:115–121

Noguchi S, Motomura K, Inaji H, Imaoka S, Koyama H (1993) Down regulation of transforming growth factor alpha by tamoxifen in human breast cancer. Cancer 72:131–136

Okamura K, Morimoto A, Hamanaka R, Ono M, Kohno K, Uchida Y, Kuwano M (1992) A model system for tumor angiogenesis: involvement of transforming growth factor-alpha in tube formation of human microvascular endothelial cells induced by esophageal cancer cells. Biochem Biophys Res Commun 186(3):1471–1479

Patterson JS (1981) Clinical aspects and development of antiestrogen therapy: a review of the endocrine effects of tamoxifen in animals and man. J Endocrinol 89:67P–75P

Prigent SA, Lemoine NR (1992) The type 1 (EGFR-related) family of growth factor receptors and their ligands. Prog Growth Factor Res 4:1–24

Robertson JFR (1996) Oestrogen receptor- a stable phenotype in breast cancer. Br J Cancer 73:5–12

Robertson JFR, Ellis IO, Walker KJ, Nicholson RI, Robins A, Blamey RW (1991) Cellular effects of tamoxifen in primary breast cancer. Br Cancer Res Treatment 20:117–123

Sainsbury JRC, Farndon JR, Harris AL, Sherbet GV (1985) Epidermal growth factor receptors on human breast cancers. Br J Surg 72:186–188

Sharma AK, Horgan K, Douglas-Jones A, McClelland R, Gee J, Nicholson RI (1994a) Dual immunocytochemical analysis of estrogen and epidermal growth factor receptors in human breast cancer. Br J Cancer 69:1032–1037

Sharma AK, Horgan K, McClelland RA, Douglas-Jones AG, Van Agthoven T, Dossers LCJ, Nicholson RI (1994b) Dual immunohistochemical assay for oestrogen and epidermal growth factor receptors in tumour cell lines. Histochem J 26:306–310

Slamon DJ, Clark GM, Wong SG et al (1987) Human breast cancer: correlation of relapse and survival with amplification of the HER-2/neu oncogene. Science 235:177–182

Staebler A, Sommer C, Mueller SC, Byers S, Thompson EW, Lupu R (1994) Modulation of breast cancer progression and differentiation by gp30/heregulin. Breast Cancer Res Treat 31:175–182

Tilly JL, Billig H, Kowalski KI, Hseuh AJ (1992) Epidermal growth factor and fibroblast growth factor suppress the spontaneous onset of apoptosis in cultured ovarian granulosa cells and follicles by a tyrosine kinase-dependent mechanism. Mol Endocrinol 6:1942–1950

Wakeling AE, Barker AJ, Davies DH, Brown DS, Green LR, Cartlidge SA, Woodburn JR (1994) Inhibition of EGF receptor tyrosine kinase activity by 4-aniloquinazolines. Br J Cancer 69 [Suppl 21]:18

Wakeling AE, Barker AJ, Davies DH, Brown DS, Green LR, Cartlidge SA, Woodburn JR (1996) Specific inhibition of epidermal growth factor receptor tyrosine kinase by 4-aniloquinazolines. Breast Cancer Res Treat 38:67–73

Walker KJ, Price-Thomas JM, Candlish W, Nicholson RI (1991) Influence of the antiestrogen tamoxifen on normal breast tissue. Br J Cancer 64:764–768

Walker RA, Varley JM (1993) The molecular pathology of human breast cancer. Cancer Surv 16:31–57

7 The Role of Estrogen in the Regulation of EGFR Expression*

R.I. Yarden, M.A. Wilson, M. Barth, and S.A. Chrysogelos

* Portions of the data in this chapter are reprinted with the permission of the publisher from R.I. Yarden, A.H. Lauber, D. El-Ashry, and S.A. Chrysogelos. Bimodel regulation of EGF receptor regulation by estrogen in breast cancer cells. Endocrinology 137(7):2739–275´47, 1996. © The Endocrine Society

7.1 Introduction

In breast cancer, epidermal growth factor receptor (EGFR) expression is inversely correlated with expression of estrogen receptor (ER) (Fitzpatrick et al. 1984; Sainsbury et al. 1985; Koenders et al. 1991; Sharma et al. 1992). While expression of ER usually predicts for responsiveness to endocrine therapy and overall good prognosis (Osborne et al. 1980), EGFR expression (independent of ER) correlates with lack of response to endocrine therapy, high incidence of metastasis, and poor survival (Koenders et al. 1991; Toi et al. 1991; Nicholson et al. 1994; Fox et al. 1994). This raises the possibility that EGFR provides an alternative growth pathway that cells are able to utilize in the absence of estrogen. An inverse correlation between ER and EGFR expression is also found in breast cancer cell lines, with ER-positive breast cancer cells expressing very low levels of EGFR (Davidson et al. 1987). Moreover, many cell regulators such as EGF, 12-*O*-tetradecanoyl phorbol acetate (TPA), and sodium butyrate have opposite effects on the expression of the two receptors (Lee et al. 1989; Secada et al. 1991; De Fazio et al. 1992). This well-established inverse correlation between EGFR and ER expression led us to hypothesize that estrogen may play an active role in maintaining low levels of EGFR expression in ER-positive breast cancer cells.

7.2 Results

7.2.1 Estrogen Withdrawal Increases Levels of EGFR mRNA and Protein

To determine if estrogen is involved in suppression of EGFR expression in ER-positive breast cancer cells, we measured changes in EGFR mRNA levels in response to estrogen withdrawal in three ER-positive breast cancer cells lines: MCF-7, T47D, and BT474. Cells were depleted of estrogen over 5 days by replacing the culture media (improved minimum essential media, IMEM, supplemented with 10% fetal bovine serum, FBS) daily with phenol red-free IMEM supplemented with 10%

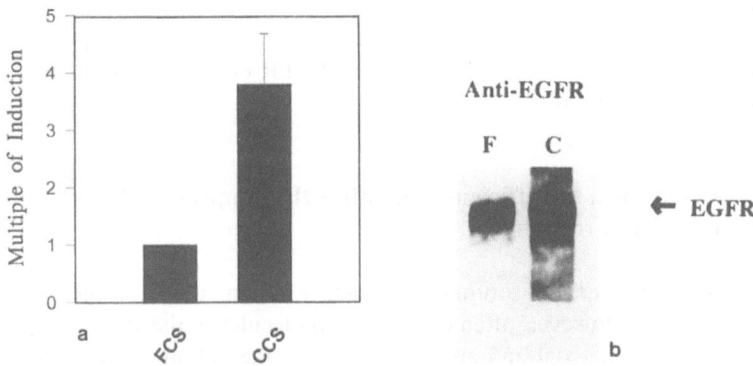

Fig. 1a,b. Effect of estrogen withdrawal on epidermal growth factor receptor (EGFR). Depletion of estrogen upregulates EGFR mRNA and protein. Estrogen receptor-positive BT474 breast cancer cells were depleted of estrogen and maintained in phenol red-free IMEM supplemented with 10% charcoal-treated calf serum (*CCS*; *C* in **b**) for 5 days or were maintained in the continuous presence of IMEM supplemented with 10% complete serum (*FCS*; fetal calf serum; *F* in **b**). **a** Cells were harvested and total RNA was isolated and analyzed by RNase protection assay using ^{32}P-labeled antisense RNA probes for EGFR and an internal control, 36B4. Autoradiograms were quantified by densitometry and EGFR values were normalized to 36B4. **b** Membrane fractions were prepared, and 100 µg of protein from each sample were electrophoresed in a 7.5% sodium dodecyl sulfate polyacrylamide gel electrophoresis (SDS-PAGE) gel transferred to a nitrocellulose membrane and then probed with the polyclonal antibody 1005 against EGFR

charcoal-treated serum (CCS). Levels of EGFR and 36B4 mRNA in estrogen-depleted cells and cells that were maintained in the presence of FBS were analyzed by RNase protection assay. The results in Fig. 1a show that in BT474 cells there is an increase in the level of EGFR mRNA in response to estrogen withdrawal. In all three breast cancer cell lines an increase of three- to sixfold in EGFR mRNA levels was determined when levels of EGFR mRNA were normalized to the level of mRNA for the ribosomal protein 36B4, which is not regulated by estrogen (Masiakowski et al. 1982). To determine whether this increase is also reflected in the amount of the receptor expressed on the cell surface we employed Western blot analysis. The membrane fractions from BT474 cells maintained in the presence of estrogen or depleted of estrogen were probed with a polyclonal antibody, 1005, directed against EGFR. As shown in Fig. 1b, the level of EGFR protein also increased in response to estrogen withdrawal, coinciding with the RNA data. This increase in EGFR mRNA and protein levels suggests that the presence of estrogen in the media can suppress EGFR expression (Yarden and Chrysogelos 1995).

7.2.2 Estrogen Is Sufficient to Mediate the Suppressive Effect on EGFR Expression

Charcoal treatment of serum is a frequently used method to deplete cells of estrogen. However, often other small molecules in the serum bind to the dextran-charcoal and are removed from the culture media by this treatment. Therefore, to specifically verify the role of estrogen in the suppression of EGFR expression, two different approaches were undertaken. First, the normal growth media of BT474 cells (IMEM supplemented with 10% FBS) was replaced with phenol-red free IMEM supplemented with 10% CCS and $10^{-8}M$ 17β-estradiol (E_2). Second, BT474 cells cultured in IMEM supplemented with 10% FBS were treated with the antiestrogens 4-hydroxytamoxifen (a partial agonist of ER) or ICI 164,384 (a pure antagonist) to specifically block estrogen action and mimic the effect of estrogen withdrawal. These conditions allow the effect of estrogen on EGFR expression to be evaluated separately from the effect of other components that might have been eliminated from the serum by the charcoal treatment. When BT474 cells were cultured in phenol red free-IMEM supplemented with both 10% CCS and E_2, EGFR mRNA did not increase, remaining at the low level found in cells cultured in IMEM supplemented with 10% FBS. When these cells were treated with antiestrogens in the presence of FBS, the level of EGFR mRNA was increased similarly to when cells were depleted of estrogen by the charcoal treatment of the serum. Both approaches indicate that the presence of estrogen alone is sufficient to suppress the expression of EGFR in ER-positive breast cancer cells (Yarden and Chrysogelos 1995).

We then asked how EGFR levels would be affected when E_2 was added back to the culture. The simplest scenario is that the addition of estrogen causes a decrease in EGFR mRNA levels back to their basal level in the presence of 10% FBS. However, it was previously reported (Mukku and Stancel 1985) that in the rat uterus estrogen can induce EGFR levels in a transient manner. Therefore, to determine whether estrogen can have differential effects on EGFR expression we have divided our study into two parts: the short-term and the long-term effects that the addition of E_2 has on EGFR expression and function.

7.2.3 Short-Term Effects of Estrogen on EGFR RNA Levels

To determine whether estrogen can induce EGFR expression in breast cancer cells as it can in the rat uterus, we studied changes in EGFR mRNA in response to E_2 in the same ER-positive cell lines (Yarden et al. 1996). Cells were depleted of estrogens over several days as described above and then treated with $10^{-8}M$ E_2 for various times up to 24 h. Figure 2a shows that in BT474 cells the level of EGFR mRNA is transiently increased in response to E_2 as soon as 30 min, is maximal at 2 h, is decreasing by 5 h following treatment, and returns to the level seen in estrogen depleted cells by 24 h. Similar results were seen with MCF-7 and T47D cells, with a maximal induction of two- to threefold at 2 h in all ER-positive cell lines tested. These data indicate that EGFR mRNA can be induced by E_2, and the rapid response may suggest a direct action mediated by ER. These results are in good agreement with the results of Lingham et al. (1988) which showed a three- to fourfold increase in EGFR mRNA in the rat uterus between 1 and 3 h after E_2 treatment, with a subsequent decline.

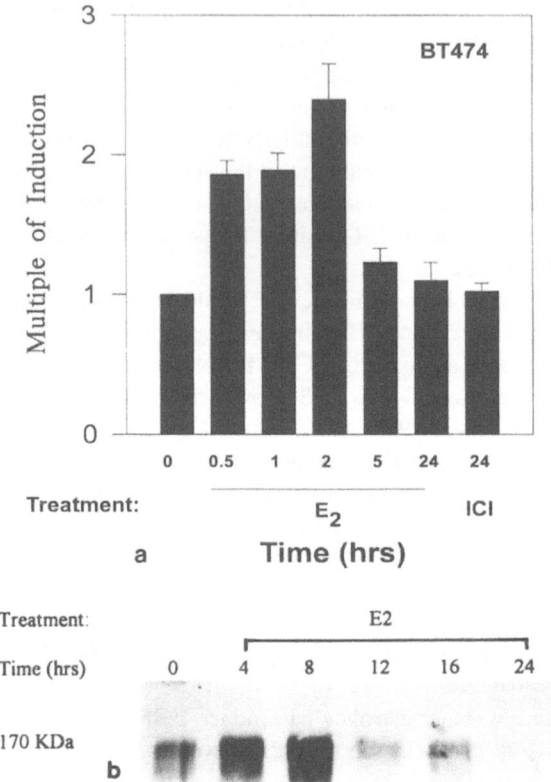

a

b

Fig. 2a,b. Short-term effect of estrogen on epidermal growth factor receptor (EGFR) mRNA and protein levels in BT474 cells. BT474 cells were depleted of estrogen and then treated with $10^{-8}M$ 17β-estradiol (*E2*). **a** Total RNA was isolated at the indicated time points and analyzed by RNase protection assay for EGFR and 36B4. Autoradiograms were quantified by scanning densitometry and values for EGFR mRNA were normalized to 36B4 mRNA in each lane and plotted as multiple of induction over control. **b** Membrane fractions were prepared, and 100 μg of protein from each sample were electrophoresed in a 7.5% sodium dodecyl sulfate polyacrylamide gel electrophoresis (SDS-PAGE) gel, transferred to a nitrocellulose membrane, and then probed with the polyclonal antibody 1005 against EGFR. (From Yarden et al. 1996)

To verify the specificity of the effect of estrogen on EGFR mRNA, BT474 cells were depleted of estrogen and then treated with E_2 for 2 h (the time point at which the maximal effect on EGFR mRNA was observed) in the absence or presence of the pure antiestrogen ICI 164,384. The results demonstrated that in the presence of E_2, EGFR mRNA levels are induced relative to untreated cells as seen before. However, this induction is completely blocked in the presence of $10^{-7}\,M$ ICI, indicating that EGFR mRNA induction is specific to estrogen and mediated by ER.

7.2.4 Effect of Estrogen on EGFR Protein Levels

To determine whether upregulation of EGFR mRNA following E_2 treatment is accompanied by an increase in EGFR protein expression, Western blot analysis with the polyclonal anti-EGFR antibody 1005 was used to detect changes in EGFR protein in response to E_2 in BT474 cells (Yarden et al. 1996). The results shown in Fig. 2b illustrate an increase in the level of EGFR protein at 4 and 8 h after treatment relative to control, estrogen-depleted cells. By 12 h, the EGFR level starts to decline, and at 24 h following E_2 addition, the level of EGFR is lower than in control cells. Overall, the EGFR response to E_2 follows the same pattern for both mRNA and protein, with a delay in protein expression relative to mRNA. This shift in the time course of the protein relative to the mRNA probably represents the time required for de novo synthesis of the receptor. The downregulation of the receptor at 24 h to levels below control may reflect both a decrease in the synthesis rate and internalization and degradation of the receptor mediated by the binding of EGFR ligands, whose expression is known to be up-regulated by estrogens (Bates et al. 1988). These results are also in agreement with those of Berthois et al. (1989), which showed a decrease in EGF binding sites when MCF-7 cells were treated with E_2 for 24 h.

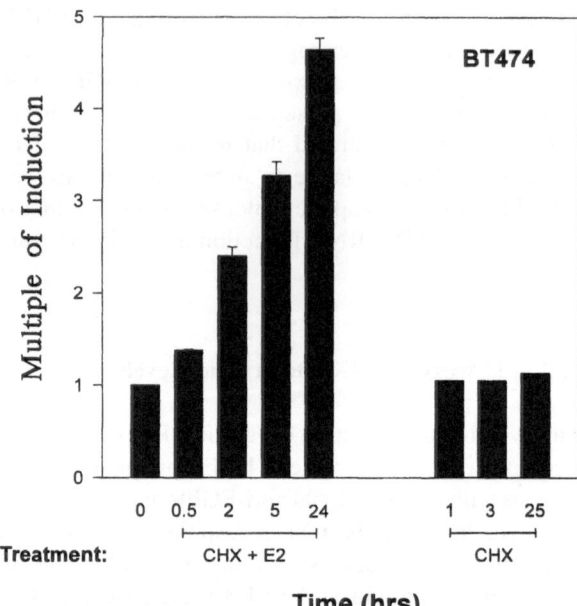

Fig. 3. Effect of cycloheximide on epidermal growth factor receptor (EGFR) mRNA in control and estrogen-treated cells. BT474 cells were depleted of estrogen and then treated with 10 μg/ml of cycloheximide (*CHX*) either 1 h prior to the addition of $10^{-8}M$ 17β-estradiol or with cycloheximide alone. Total RNA was prepared from cells harvested at the indicated time points following addition of estradiol (*E2*), and analyzed for EGFR and 36B4 by RNase protection assay. Autoradiograms were quantified by scanning densitometry and normalized values of EGFR mRNA were plotted as multiple of induction relative to control, estrogen depleted cells. (From Yarden et al. 1996)

7.2.5 Role of Protein Synthesis in Estrogen Regulation: Effect of Cycloheximide on EGFR mRNA Expression

In order to determine whether E_2 acts directly on the EGFR gene or requires the synthesis of other proteins, we investigated the effect of the protein synthesis inhibitor cycloheximide on the induction of EGFR mRNA by E_2 in MCF-7 and BT474 cells (Yarden et al. 1996). Cycloheximide alone did not result in induction of EGFR mRNA levels at 1-,

Table 1. Induction of EGFR mRNA in ER+ breast cancer cells following estrogen treatment

Treatment	Multiple of induction	
	2 h	24 h
Estrogen	1.5–2.5	1
Estrogen + cycloheximide	1.5–2.5	2.5–5

3-, or 25-h treatment as shown in Fig. 3 for BT474 cells. Treatment with cycloheximide 1 h prior to the addition of $10^{-8} M$ E_2 to MCF-7 or BT474 cells did not abolish EGFR mRNA upregulation as measured by RNase protection relative to 36B4 mRNA. A 1.5- to 2.5-fold induction of EGFR mRNA was seen in both cell lines after 2 h of E_2 treatment, equivalent to the fold induction that was observed in the absence of cycloheximide. However, the presence of cycloheximide together with E_2 inhibited the EGFR mRNA downregulation that was previously seen after 5 h of E_2 treatment alone. In the presence of both cycloheximide and E_2, EGFR mRNA levels continued to increase, up to fivefold at 24 h in BT474 cells (Fig. 3), and 2.5-fold in MCF-7 cells relative to control, estrogen-depleted cells, as summarized in Table 1. Thus, the increase in EGFR mRNA within 2 h of E_2 treatment is independent of protein synthesis, pointing to a direct effect of ER on the EGFR gene, whereas the subsequent downregulation of EGFR mRNA does require de novo protein synthesis, suggesting the involvement of a protein or proteins, such as a repressor or nuclease, that functions to maintain low levels of EGFR expression in the presence of estrogen.

7.2.6 mRNA Stability Is Not Involved in Estrogen Regulation of EGFR

While the results of the cycloheximide experiments suggest a direct transcriptional effect of estrogen on EGFR levels, it is possible that posttranscriptional regulation also plays a role. To investigate the involvement of mRNA stability as a mechanism that controls EGFR mRNA expression, we first measured the steady state half-life of EGFR mRNA in MCF-7, T47D, and BT474 ER-positive breast cancer cells.

These studies were carried out by the addition of the transcription inhibitor actinomycin D at 5 µg/ml to the cells and analysis of the rate of EGFR mRNA decay by RNase protection assay. In all ER-positive cell lines used in this study we have found that the half-life of EGFR mRNA is approximately 1 h. A half-life of 1 h for EGFR mRNA has also been reported in A431 and in MDA-468 cell lines (Jinno et al. 1988; Hamburger and Pinnamaneni 1991). We then measured the half-life of EGFR mRNA in BT474 cells that were depleted of estrogen, and in cells that were treated with E_2 for 1 h or 3.5 h prior to the addition of actinomycin D to determine whether changes seen in EGFR mRNA levels in response to E_2 (either the induction or subsequent downregulation) are due to alterations in EGFR mRNA stability. No changes were found in EGFR mRNA half-life under any of these conditions, implicating transcriptional control as the primary mechanism involved in alterations in EGFR expression in response to estrogen (Yarden et al. 1996).

7.2.7 Estrogen Induces EGFR Gene Transcription

The above results strongly suggest transcription as the main mechanism that controls EGFR expression in response to E_2. To directly test this, we performed nuclear run-on assays. In these experiments BT474 cells were treated with E_2 and nuclei were isolated at subsequent time points. Both a 3.8-kb, full-length cDNA of EGFR and a genomic fragment containing the 5' untranslated region of the EGFR gene and the first exon were used as probes to detect EGFR gene transcription. A rapid and transient transcriptional increase of three- to fourfold relative to untreated cells was observed at 2 h following E_2 addition for both 5'-EGFR and EGFR cDNA. This increase was followed by a dramatic decrease in EGFR gene transcription, returning to the basal level as soon as 5 h following E_2 addition and remaining at that level at 24 h (Yarden et al. 1996). These results are in good agreement with our results obtained for EGFR mRNA levels and clearly indicate that both up- and downregulation of EGFR mRNA in response to estrogen are under transcriptional control.

7.2.8 Putative Estrogen Responsive Elements in the EGFR Promoter

Since estrogen is known to mediate transcription through specific sequences called estrogen responsive elements (EREs) we wished to determine the existence of these sequences in the 5'-flanking region of the EGFR gene. It is important to note that to date the EGFR promoter region had been sequenced from two different sources by two different groups (Ishii et al. 1985; Haley et al. 1987), and there are several

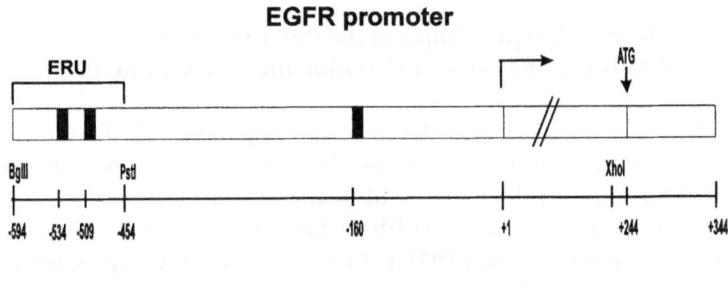

EGFR promoter

■ Putative ERE

Putative EREs

Position	Sequence
-534 to -523	GGGCAnnnCGACC
-509 to -495	GGCCAnnnnnTGATC
-160 to -148	GGCCAnnnTGTCC
Consensus ERE:	**GGTCAnnnTGACC**

Fig. 4. Schematic diagram of the EGFR promoter and the putative estrogen responsive elements (*ERE*) sequences. The position of the putative EREs is shown relative to the major in vivo transcription start site and relevant restriction sites. The estrogen-responsive unit (*ERU*) that was used for electrophoresis mobility shift assays (EMSAs) is composed of the two imperfect palindromes that reside between positions –534 and –495 and are separated by 14 bp. The third putative response element resides between positions –160 to –148. The consensus ERE sequence is also shown for comparison.(From Yarden et al. 1996)

discrepancies between the two published sequences. Therefore, we sequenced a 840-bp *Bgl*II-*Xho*I fragment that contains the proximal EGFR promoter from human fetal liver. Scanning the promoter sequence revealed no consensus EREs; however, three imperfect palindromes with one base pair change in each half-site were identified (Yarden et al. 1996). These imperfect palindromes are located at positions −534 to −523, −509 to −495 and −160 to −148 relative to the major transcription start site, as shown in Fig. 4. The sequence of each of these putative EREs compared to the consensus ERE is also shown.

7.2.9 Estrogen Receptor Binds to the Putative EREs Located Between −534 and −495 Within the EGFR Promoter

To determine whether the ER can form complexes with the putative EREs identified, electrophoresis mobility shift assays (EMSA) were carried out using a 138-bp *Xba*I-*Pst*I fragment from the EGFR promoter that contains the two imperfect EREs that are separated by 14 bp (the estrogen-responsive unit, ERU) and a yeast extract overexpressing recombinant human ER (Yarden et al. 1996). A retarded band was observed in the presence of the human ER (hER) that was supershifted with the antibody h151 directed against the hinge region of the ER. When a 130-bp fragment consisting of two perfect EREs separated by 21 bp was used as a positive control, we also observed a shifted band that could be further supershifted in the presence of the h151 anti-ER antibody, as expected; however, these bands migrated faster than those formed with the fragment of the EGFR promoter. No complexes were formed with a nonsense fragment where the specific base composition was maintained but the sequence was rearranged so that no palindromes were present.

7.2.10 Estrogen Induces EGFR Gene Transcription via Imperfect Response Elements in the EGFR Promoter Region

Since we found that estrogen induces EGFR transcription and there are putative EREs in the EGFR promoter region that can be bound by ER, we wished to confirm that the promoter region can drive transcription of a reporter gene in response to estrogen and, furthermore, determine the involvement of the putative elements in this induction. Therefore, we constructed reporter gene constructs where we placed upstream of the luciferase gene either the 840 bp of the proximal promoter or a mutated promoter in which the 140 bp ERU region was replaced by a nonsense sequence of the same size (Fig. 5a). A construct containing two consensus EREs in the context of mouse mammary tumor virus-long terminal repeat (MMTV-LTR) driving the luciferase gene was used as a positive control for estrogen induction and a promoterless construct was used as a control for background activity of the enzyme. The constructs were transfected by the lipofectamine method into MCF-7 cells that were rapidly depleted of estrogen, and the following day the cells were treated with 10^{-8} M E_2 or 10^{-7} M ICI or left untreated for 30 h. The results from the luciferase assay as shown in Fig. 5b demonstrate E_2-induced luciferase activity of the EGFR promoter relative to ICI-treated or untreated cells. Removal of the putative ERU region from the EGFR promoter eliminated the E_2-induced activity, indicating that estrogen induction of EGFR is mediated through the promoter region and, more specifically, via the ERU region. The consensus EREs gave, as expected, strong estrogenic induction as measured by luciferase activity.

7.2.11 Prolonged Presence of Estrogen Suppresses the Level of EGFR mRNA

Our original observation was that estrogen depletion of ER-positive breast cancer cells results in the induction of EGFR mRNA levels. Upon treatment of estrogen-depleted ER-positive breast cancer cells with E_2 there is a further two- to threefold transient increase in EGFR mRNA levels and both this increase and the subsequent downregulation following E_2 addition are rapid, resulting at 24 h post E_2 addition in the plateauing of EGFR mRNA levels at the same level as in estrogen-depleted cells. Since EGFR mRNA levels in cells maintained in FBS are lower than this plateau reached at 24 h of E_2 treatment, we speculated that the long-term presence of estrogen is responsible for the low levels of EGFR expression in cells maintained in FBS. Therefore, we depleted BT474 cells of estrogen, and then added back 10^{-8} M E_2 to phenol-red-free IMEM supplemented with 10% CCS for various times.

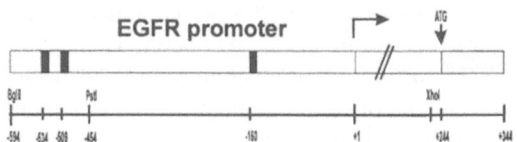

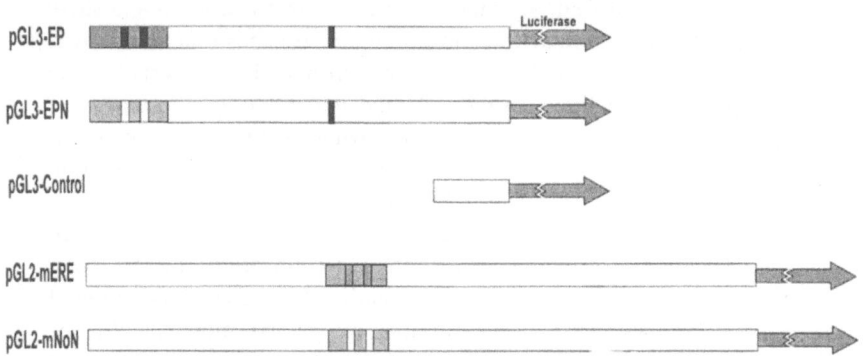

a   ▮ Putative ERE ▮ ERE ▯ NON ▭▷ Luciferase gene

Fig. 5a,b. The epidermal growth factor receptor *(EGFR)* estrogen-responsive unit *(ERU)* can mediate estrogen induction of a reporter gene in a transient transfection assay. **a** Reporter gene constructs: the endogenous EGFR promoter and first exon is shown at the top, with the wild-type *(pGL3-EP)* and mutated *(pGL3-EPN)* EGFR promoters linked to the luciferase reporter gene of the promoterless expression vector pGL3 displayed below. The positive *(pGL2-mERE)* and negative *(pGL2-mNON)* control constructs which consist of the mouse mammary tumor virus-long terminal repeat (MMTV-LTR) with either consensus estrogen-responsive element *(ERE)* or nonsense sequence (inserted in the unique *Bgl*II site) linked to the luciferase reporter gene are also shown. **b** see p. 143

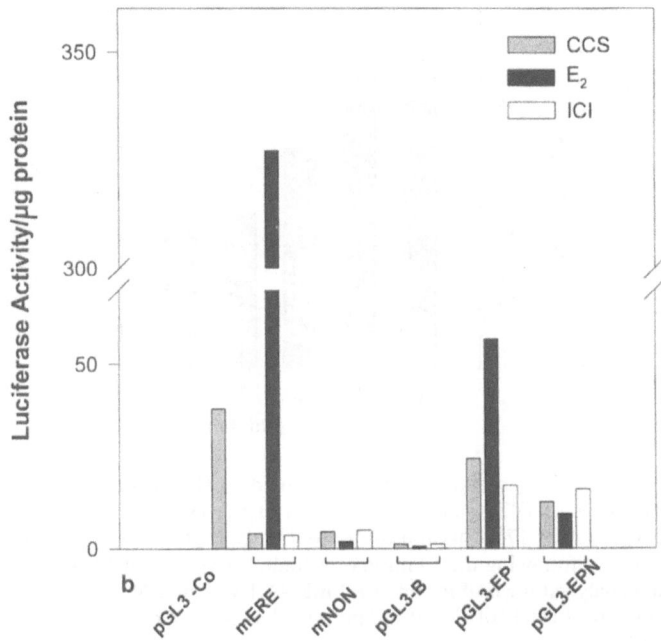

Fig. 5b. Transient transfection assays were performed in MCF-7 cells that were rapidly depleted of estrogen; 16 h after transfection of 10 μg plasmid DNA into the cells by the lipofectamine method, the culture media was replaced and cells were treated with $10^{-8}M$ estradiol (E_2) or $10^{-7}M$ *ICI* for 30 h as indicated. Luciferase activity is corrected for background light emission and protein concentration of the extracts. *CCS*, charcoal-treated serum; pGL3-B is the promoterless lucierferase vector control; pGL3-Co contains the SV40 promoter and enhancer and is a positive luciferase control; mERE and mNON are positive and negative controls, respectively, for estrogen response

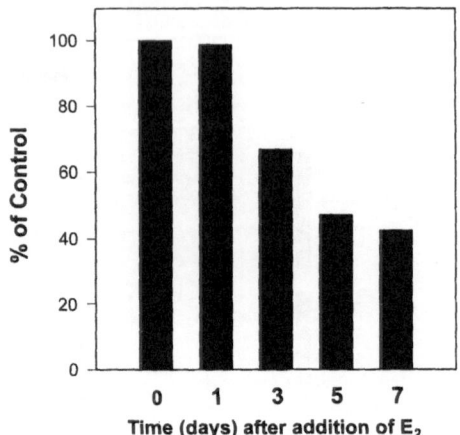

Fig. 6. Long-term estrogen downregulates epidermal growth factor receptor (EGFR) mRNA. BT474 cells were depleted of estrogen for 5 days and then treated with $10^{-8}M$ 17β-estradiol for up to 7 days. Cells were harvested at the indicated days following the addition of estradiol (E_2), and total RNA was isolated and analyzed for EGFR and 36B4 mRNA levels by RNase protection assay. Normalized levels of EGFR are presented as percent of control, estrogen-depleted cells

RNA was extracted from cells at the times indicated in Fig. 6, analyzed by RNase protection assay, and EGFR mRNA levels were normalized to levels of 36B4 RNA. The results shown in Fig. 6 reveal a gradual decrease in EGFR mRNA levels starting at day 3 following addition of E_2. At 7 days of E_2 treatment, EGFR mRNA decreased to 40% of the level in estrogen-depleted cells, a level similar to that previously observed in cells maintained in the presence of FBS. These results indicate that the long-term presence of estrogen has a suppressive effect on EGFR expression.

7.2.12 Estrogen Suppression of EGFR
Is at the Transcriptional Level

Previously, we had found that the half-life of EGFR mRNA was 1 h in either the presence or absence of estrogen, strongly suggesting that changes in EGFR mRNA stability do not contribute to the difference we have observed in the level of EGFR expression. We therefore investigated the role of transcription as the mechanism of suppression using a nuclear run-on assay with nuclei isolated from BT474 cells maintained in FBS or depleted of estrogen. While transcription of the progesterone receptor and pS2 genes was reduced threefold, estrogen withdrawal resulted in a two-to threefold increase in EGFR gene transcription. These results are in good agreement with our findings for EGFR mRNA levels and clearly indicate that removal of estrogen results in transcriptional upregulation of the EGFR gene.

7.2.13 Estrogen Depleted Cells Are More Responsive
to Growth Factors

To address whether the increase in EGFR levels in estrogen-depleted cells sensitizes these cells to low levels of growth factors and thus provides an alternative pathway for growth, we performed growth assays that tested the ability of EGF to affect cell proliferation. BT474 cells were cultured in IMEM supplemented with 10% FBS or in phenol red-free IMEM supplemented with 10% CCS plus or minus $10^{-8}\,M$ $E_2 \cdot$EGF at a concentration of $10^{-8}\,M$ was assessed for the ability to increase cell growth under these different culture conditions. In the absence of estrogen, EGF had a much stronger proliferative effect (Table 2), indicating that estrogen-depleted cells (which express higher levels of EGFR on their surface) are more sensitive to EGFR ligands. To further address this hypothesis, we performed similar growth assays with EGF in which BT474 cells were cultured in IMEM supplemented with 10% FBS and the antiestrogens ICI 164,384 or 4-hydroxytamoxifen. Treatment with these antiestrogens results in cell growth arrest and an increase in EGFR expression. EGF was able to induce cell growth under these conditions again suggesting that estrogen-depleted cells have a higher sensitivity to EGFR ligands and that signaling

Table 2. Effect of EGF on BT474 cell growth

Growth	% Untreated cells	
Conditions	6 days	9 days
FBS	133	–
$CCS + E_2$	143	142
CCS	160	219
FBS + Tam	227	–
FBS + ICI	196	284[a]

BT474 cells were plated at 500 cells/well supplemented with 10% fetal bovine serum (FBS) in the presence or absence of $10^{-7}M$ ICI or $5\times10^{-7}M$ 4-hydroxy tamoxifen or with 10% charcoal-treated serum (CCS) in the presence or absence of estrogen. Human recombinant epidermal growth factor (EGF) was added at $10^{-8}M$ to the cells (with each treatment consisting of ten replicates) on the following day. Cells were harvested at the indicated times, stained with crystal violet, and relative growth was measured by light emission at 540 nm and expressed as the percent of control untreated cells for the given time point.
[a] Time point is 8 days.

through EGFR can provide these cells with an alternative growth pathway.

The clinical implications of these results are potentially important. We have demonstrated not only that depletion of estrogen by antiestrogens, such as tamoxifen, that are used in endocrine therapy causes an increase in the expression level of EGFR, but that it also sensitizes the cells to growth factors that provide the cells with an alternative growth pathway. Since EGFR expression in tumors correlates with advanced disease and poor survival, these results suggest that treatment with antiestrogens may contribute to the progression of breast cancer to a more aggressive phenotype, at least in part by affecting EGFR levels and signaling. Hence, it might be useful to investigate a combination of treatments for these two alternative pathways.

7.2.14 EGFR Upregulation in Response to Growth Inhibition: A Survival Mechanism in ER-Positive Breast Cancer Cells?

The above results indicate that signaling through EGFR in the absence of estrogen induces cells to re-enter the cell cycle, and can provide an alternative growth stimulation. In the absence of estrogen, the cells arrest in the G1 phase of the cell cycle. We hypothesize that the cells upregulate EGFR as a survival mechanism to avoid cell death. Therefore, the question that arises is whether blocking the two pathways simultaneously will cause the cells to undergo apoptosis. To test this hypothesis, we performed a cell death detection enzyme-linked immunosorbent assay (ELISA). The data in Fig. 7 demonstrate that depleting the cells of estrogen or blocking signaling of EGFR by itself does not result in an increase in apoptotic cell death compared to control untreated cells. However, simultaneously depleting the cells of estrogen

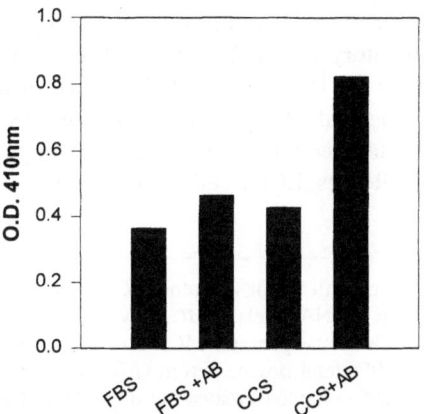

Fig. 7. Effect of estrogen withdrawal and epidermal growth factor receptor (EGFR) signaling blockade on cell death. BT474 cells were plated at 1×10^5 cells/well in six well plates. On the following day, the cells were depleted of estrogen and/or treated with 15 μg/ml of the EGFR neutralizing antibody 225IgG, as indicated. Fresh treatments were added to the cells after 48 h, and an additional 48 h later the cells were harvested. Cytoplasmic lysates were prepared and analyzed for DNA and nucleosome content by the cell death enzyme-linked immunosorbent assay (ELISA). *FBS*, fetal bovine serums; *AB*, antibody; *CCS*, charcoal-treated serum

and blocking EGFR signaling causes a twofold increase in apoptosis as detected by the presence of mono- and oligonucleosomes in the cytoplasmic fraction of the cells. These results strongly suggest that upregulation of EGFR in response to estrogen depletion is a survival mechanism the cells are inducing to avoid cell death.

7.2.15 Increased EGFR Expression in Response to Estrogen Withdrawal: A Model for Breast Cancer Progression

The results described so far indicate that in the presence of estrogen, EGFR levels are repressed. Once estrogen is removed, EGFR levels increase and the cells become more sensitive to EGFR ligands. It is a possibile that the long-term absence of estrogen will result in selection for a subpopulation of cells that express higher levels of EGFR and are less dependent on estrogen for growth since they are sensitized to low concentrations of ligands. To investigate this potential mechanism of breast cancer progression, we utilized an in vitro model system, developed by the laboratory of Dr. R. Clarke, Lombardi Cancer Center, Georgetown University (Brünner et al. 1993a,b). In this system, ER-positive, estrogen-dependent MCF-7 cells were twice selected in vivo in ovariectomized nude mice for estrogen independent growth to yield the MIII and LCC1 cell lines. LCC1 cells were then selected once more in

---

Fig. 8a,b. Epidermal growth factor receptor (EGFR) mRNA levels in MCF-7 ▶ variants cells. **a** EGFR mRNA levels in *MCF-7* variant cells were analyzed and compared to the levels in the parental MCF-7 cells cultured either in IMEM supplemented with 10% fetal bovine serum (*FBS*) or phenol-red free IMEM supplemented with 10% charcoal-treated serum (*CCS*). Total RNA was isolated from subconfluent cultures, analyzed by RNase protection assay, and EGFR mRNA levels were normalized to 36B4 mRNA. Data are represented relative to the basal level in the parental MCF-7 cells in the presence of FBS.
b The effect of estrogen on EGFR mRNA levels was analyzed in MCF-7 variant cells *MIII* and *LCC2*. Cells were cultured for 5 days in phenol red-free IMEM supplemented with 10% CCS alone or in combination with $10^{-8}M$ estradiol (E_2). RNA was isolated, analyzed by RNase protection assay, and EGFR mRNA levels were normalized to 36B4 mRNA. Data are represented relative to the basal level for each cell line when cultured under estrogen-free conditions

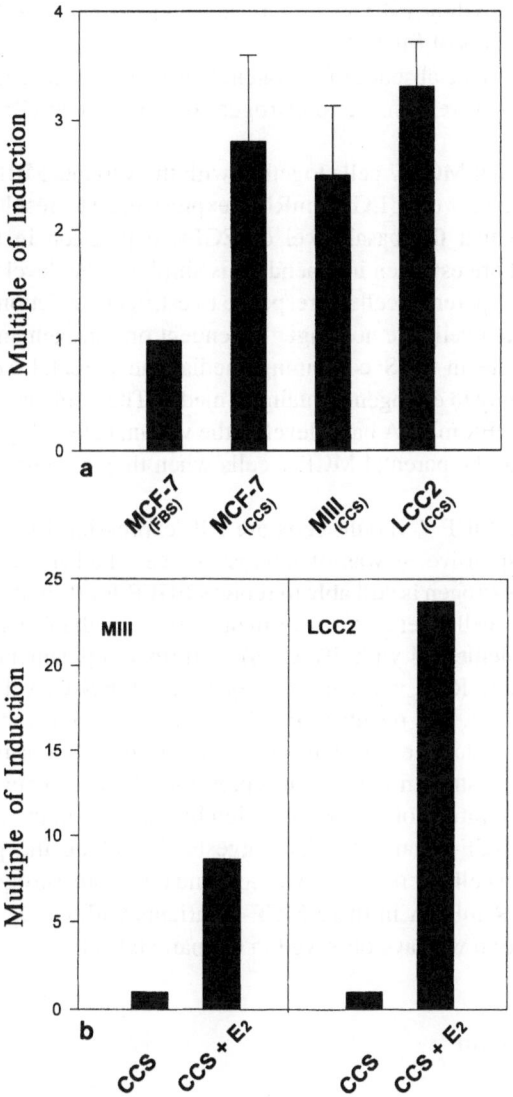

Fig. 8. Legend see p. 148

vitro for tamoxifen-resistant growth to yield the cell line LCC2. The different variants of MCF-7 are maintained permanently in CCS and are able to grow in the absence of estrogen; however, they have not lost their ER and are still responsive to estrogen to some extent (Brünner et al. 1993a,b).

The parental MCF-7 cells together with the variants MIII and LCC2 were analyzed for their EGFR mRNA expression. The results in Fig. 8a demonstrate that the basal level of EGFR expression in the MCF-7 variants that are estrogen independent is similar to the level that is seen in the MCF-7 parental cells in response to estrogen depletion. While the MCF-7 variant cells are no longer dependent on estrogen and therefore can proliferate in CCS containing media, the parental MCF-7 cells proliferate only in estrogen-containing media. The implication therefore is that the EGFR mRNA basal level of the variant cells is higher than the basal level in the parental MCF-7 cells when they are propagated continuously.

Since the MCF-7 variant cells are still expressing ER and are still estrogen responsive, it was of interest to see whether the continuous presence of estrogen is still able to repress EGFR levels in these cells. To that end, the cells were grown in their normal media (phenol red-free IMEM supplemented with 5% CCS) or further supplemented with E_2 for 5 days, and RNA was analyzed for EGFR mRNA levels by RNase protection assay. The results in Fig. 8b demonstrate again that EGFR is an estrogen inducible gene; however, additional factors must be involved in the estrogen-dependent repression of EGFR expression. The sustained magnitude of EGFR induction by estrogen in the estrogen-independent MCF-7 variant cells suggests that along the pathway of progression a cellular repressor was lost and therefore estrogen is able to induce EGFR mRNA in these MCF-7 variants without the subsequent downregulation we have observed in the parental cells.

7.3 Discussion

The inverse correlation between EGFR and ER expression in breast cancer is well established both in tumors and in cell lines; however, the mechanism responsible for this relationship is yet unknown. We have investigated the hormonal regulation of the EGF receptor in human breast cancer cells that express low levels of EGFR by analyzing the role of estrogen as a modulator of EGFR expression. In summary, we have shown that estrogen can regulate EGFR expression both positively and negatively, and the inverse correlation between EGFR and ER appears to be a result of a direct interaction between ER and the EGFR gene that forms the basis of a complex regulation mediated by estrogen. In the continuous presence of estrogen, estrogen-dependent, ER-positive breast cancer cells express low levels of EGFR, whereas in the absence of estrogen, these cells upregulate EGFR mRNA and protein levels. At the same time, the cells become sensitized to EGFR ligands, suggesting that EGFR induction may represent an attempt of the cells to survive, and in fact when the EGFR signaling pathway is blocked simultaneously with estrogen depletion, the cells undergo apoptosis.

On the molecular level, there is an increase in basal transcription of the EGFR gene in the absence of estrogen. These results imply that a transcriptional repression of EGFR expression is relieved once estrogen is removed. Estrogen itself can further induce EGFR mRNA and protein levels when added back to the culture media. However, EGFR induction is transient, and within a few hours EGFR levels return to the level found under estrogen-free conditions; it is only after long exposure to estrogen (several days) that EGFR levels return to their initial low basal level. These results indicate that estrogen regulation of EGFR is complex and occurs at multiple levels involving both inductive and repressive components. We would like to suggest a model in which a candidate repressor protein might also be regulated by estrogen. Therefore, when cells are depleted of estrogen, the repressor levels diminish and the interference with estrogen induction is lifted. However, the addition of E_2 results in its synthesis over a longer time course than EGFR. Thus, only a limited increase in EGFR is observed before sufficient amounts of the repressor have been synthesized.

Taken together with the known inverse correlation between ER and EGFR in breast cancer, our results have intriguing implications for breast cancer progression. As breast cancer progresses, tumors often lose their estrogen dependence, and EGFR is upregulated. One can suggest a role for upregulation of EGFR first as a survival mechanism for the cells and ultimately to provide an alternative, estrogen-independent pathway for growth. Similarly, treatment of breast cancer with antiestrogenic drugs could give rise to a population of cells with increased levels of EGFR expression that ultimately can bypass the requirement for estrogen and become hormone independent and nonresponsive to treatment.

Acknowledgments. The authors wish to thank Dr. Dorraya El-Ashry, Dr. Michael Johnson, and Dr. Marc Lippman for many helpful discussions. The yeast extracts expressing the human ER were kindly provided by Dr. N. Weigel, Baylor College of Medicine, antibody h151 directed against the hinge region of the human ER was the kind gift of Dr. D. Edwards, University of Colorado Health Sciences Center, and the EGFR blocking antibody 225 was generously provided by Dr. H. Masui, Memorial Sloan-Kettering Cancer Center. This work was supported by a grant from the National Cancer Institute (CA55677) to S. Chrysogelos, and in part by the Lombardi Cancer Center Tissue Culture Core Facility, U.S. Public Health Service Grant 2P30-CA51008 and SPORE Grant 2P50-CA58185.

References

Bates SB, Davidson NE, Valverius EM, Freter CE, Dickson RB, Tam JP, Kudlow JE, Lippman ME, Salomon DS (1988) Expression of transforming growth factor-α and its messenger RNa in human breast cancer: its regulation by estrogen and its possible functional significance. Mol Endocrinol 2:543–555

Berthois Y, Dong XF, Martin PM (1989) Regulation of epidermal growth factor-receptor by estrogen and antiestrogen in the human breast cancer cell line MCF-7. Biochem Biophys Res Commun 159:126–131

Brünner N, Boulay V, Fojo A, Freter CE, Lippman ME, Clarke R (1993a) Acquisition of hormone independent growth in MCF-7 cells is accompanied by increased expression of estrogen-regulated genes but without detectable DNA amplification. Cancer Res 53:283–290

Brünner N, Fransden TL, Holst-Hansen C, Bei M, Thompson EW, Wakeling AE, Lippman ME, Clarke R (1993b) MCF-7-LCC2: a 4-hydroxytamoxifen resistant human breast cancer variant that retains sensetivity to the steroidal antiestrogen ICI 182,780. Cancer Res 53:3229–3232

Davidson NE, Gelmann EP, Lippman ME, Dickson RB (1987) Epidermal growth factor receptor gene expression in estrogen positive and negative human breast cancer cell lines. Mol Endocrinol 1:216–223

De Fazio A, Chiew Y-E, Donoghue C, Lee CSL, Sutherland RL (1992) Effect of sodium butyrate or estrogen receptor and epidermal growth factor receptor gene expression in human breast cancer cell lines. J Biol Chem 267:18008–18012

Fitzpatrick SL, Brightwell J, Wittliff JL, Barrows GH, Schultz GS (1984) Epidermal growth factor binding by breast tumor biopsies and relationship to estrogen and progestin receptor levels. Cancer Res 44:3448–3453

Fox SB, Smith K, Hollyer J, Greenall M, Hastrich D, Harris AL (1994) The epidermal growth factor receptor as a prognostic marker: results of 370 patients and review of 3009 patients. Breast Cancer Res Treat 29:41–49

Haley J, Whittle N, Bennett P, Kinchington D, Ullrich A, Waterfield M (1987) The human EGF receptor gene: structure of 110 Kb locus and identification of sequences regulating its transcription. Oncogene Res 1:375–396

Hamburger AW, Pinnamaneni GD (1991) Increased epidermal growth factor receptor gene expression by γ-interferon in a human breast carcinoma cell line. Br J Cancer 64:64–68

Ishii S, Xu Y-H, Stratton RH, Roe BA, Merlino GT, Pastan I (1985) Characterization and sequence of the promoter region of the human epidermal growth factor receptor gene. Proc Natl Acad Sci USA 82:4920–4924

Jinno Y, Merlino GT, Pastan I (1988) A novel effect of EGF on mRNA stability. Nucleic Acids Res 16:4975–4966

Koenders PG, Beex LVAM, Geurts-Moespot A, Heuvel JJTM, Kienhuis CBM, Benraad TJ (1991) Epidermal growth factor receptor-negative tumors are predominantly confined to the subgroup of estradiol receptor-positive human primary breast cancer. Cancer Res 51:4544–4548

Lee CSL, Koga M, Sutherland RL (1989) Modulation of estrogen receptor and epidermal growth factor receptor mRNA by phorbol ester in MCF-7 breast cancer cells. Biochem Biophys Res Commun 162:415–421

Lingham RB, Stancel GM, Loose-Mitchell DS (1988) Estrogen regulation of epidermal growth factor receptor messenger ribonucleic acid. Mol Endocrinol 2:230–235

Masiakowski P, Breathnach R, Bloch J, Gannon F, Krust A, Chambon P (1982) Cloning of cDNA sequences of hormone regulated genes from the MCF-7 human breast cancer cell line. Nucleic Acids Res 10:7895–7903

Mukku VR, Stancel GM (1985) Regulation of epidermal growth factor receptor by estrogen. J Biol Chem 260:9820–9824

Nicholson RI, McClelland R, Gee JMW, Manning DL, Cannnon P, Robertson JFR, Ellis IO, Blamey RW (1994) Epidermal growth factor receptor expression in breast cancer: association with reasponse to endocrine therapy. Breast Cancer Res Treat 29:117–126

Osborne CK, Yochmowitz MG, Knight WA III, McGuire WL (1980) The value of estrogen and progesterone receptors in the treatment of breast cancer. Cancer 46:2884–2888

Sainsbury JRC, Frandon JR, Sherbet GV, Harris AL (1985) Epidermal growth factor receptors and estrogen receptors in human breast cancer. Lancet i:364–366

Secada M, Knabbe C, Dickson RB, Lippman ME, Bronzert D, Lindsey RK, Gottardis MM, Martin MB (1991) Post-transcriptional destabilization of estrogen receptor mRNA in MCF-7 cells by 12-O-tetradecanoylphorbol-13 acetate. J Biol Chem 266:17809–17814

Sharma AK, Horgan K, Douglas-Joanes AG, McClelland RA, Nicholson RI (1992) Double immunohistochemical assay of receptors for estrogen (ER) and epidermal growth factor (EGFR). Breast Cancer Res Treat 23:185

Toi M, Osaki A, Yamada H, Toge T (1991) Epidermal growth factor receptor expression as a prognostic indicator in breast cancer. Eur J Cancer 27:977–980

Yarden RI, Chrysogelos SA (1995) Estrogen mediated suppression of EGFR expression in estrogen responsive breast cancer cells. J Cell Biochem 19A:46

Yarden RI, Lauber AH, El-Ashry D, Chrysogelos SA (1996) Bimodal regulation of EGF receptor regulation by estrogen in breast cancer cells. Endocrinology 137:2739–2747

8 Multifunctional Growth Factors in Tumor Progression

F. Radvanyi, S. Bellusci, B. Boyer, J. Jouanneau, P. Savagner,
A.M. Vallés, and J.P. Thiery

8.1 In Vitro Studies of Epithelial Cell Plasticity: The NBT-II Model

Our goal is to analyze the role of multifunctional growth factors in epithelial plasticity and, specifically, to study the contribution of these factors to the loss of cohesion among tumor cells leading to the acquisition of motile, invasive, and metastatic behavior.

Our studies in the past years focused on a rat bladder carcinoma cell line NBT-II (Toyoshima et al. 1971). In vitro, this cell line can switch from an epithelial, nonmotile state, to a dispersed, motile, mesenchymal-like state. This transition can be triggered experimentally by plating cells or aggregates on several collagen types or by adding different growth factors to the culture medium (Tchao 1982; Boyer et al. 1989a; Tucker et al. 1990, 1991a; Vallés et al. 1990a). The rapid induction of the transition, which can be reversed upon removal of the inducers, provides a suitable model to study mechanisms controlling the stability of epithelial cell organization. The progression of carcinoma is often accompanied by a dedifferentiation of the epithelial cells, including the loss of well-defined junctional complexes. During embryonic development, transient or permanent conversions of epithelial tissues to a mesenchymal state allows morphogenesis to proceed towards more elaborated structures, particularly through inductive events which occur in time and space between mesenchyme and their closely associated epithelia. This process, designated epithelial–mesenchymal transition (EMT), has been well described during gastrulation of several vertebrates, in the ontogeny of the neural crest in all vertebrates, and in somite differentiation. By analogy, we will also call the conversion observed in NBT-II cells an EMT. The NBT-II model is not unique as there are other examples of cell lines which are able to scatter in response to a growth factor; for example, MDCK cells, which have an epithelial phenotype, respond to HGF/SF (hepatocyte growth factor, also called scatter factor) by cell scattering (Nakamura et al. 1989; Weidner et al. 1990, 1991). Epidermal growth factor (EGF) and transforming growth factor-α (TGF-α) induce morphological changes in an immortalized human mammary epithelial cell line 184A1. In contrast to the NBT-II cells, this effect is transient: after 3 days of exposure to EGF, the cells downregulate their EGF receptors and return to the epithelial state (Matthay et al. 1993).

8.1.1 Growth Factors Induced EMT in NBT-II Cells

The EMT of NBT-II cells involves the loss of a well-defined epithelial organization, including the disruption of junctional complexes. The resulting individual cells assume a spindle-like fibroblastoid appearance and become motile, as revealed by time-lapse videomicroscopy (Boyer et al. 1989a,b). Several growth factors (fibroblast growth factor 1/acidic fibroblast growth factor, FGF-1/aFGF; EGF; TGF-α; HGF/SF) are able to induce the EMT of NBT-II cells (Bellusci et al. 1994a; Gavrilovic et al. 1990; Vallés et al. 1990a). All these growth factors share the common property of activating tyrosine kinase receptors. Tyrosine kinase inhibitors such as tyrphostins or genistein abrogate the scattering activity of growth factors.

8.1.2 The Response to Growth Factors Depends on Cell Density

We have discovered that NBT-II cells exhibit two completely different responses to growth factors (Vallés et al. 1990b). At low cell density, growth factors such as FGF-1 act as scattering agents that can convert the epithelial NBT-II cells into fibroblastic-like, motile cells. Under these conditions, NBT-II cells are unresponsive to the mitogenic effects of FGF-1. At high cell density, FGF-1 is a potent mitogenic factor but its scattering activity is essentially abrogated. Slight modifications in the binding of FGF-1 to its receptors are observed at high cell density, which correlate with a downregulation of receptors with no apparent change in their molecular form. NBT-II cells located at the edge of artificial wounds mimic the behavior of subconfluent cells, since they undergo an EMT and do not proliferate upon FGF-1 treatment. Furthermore, in large-sized NBT-II colonies, peripheral cells are the first to dissociate in response to FGF-1. Altogether, our results suggest that the cellular response to multifunctional growth factors might depend on the position of the cell within the responding cell population. It is likely that the same FGF receptor (FGFR2b) (Savagner et al. 1994) trigger these two distinct responses and thus it appears that cells in a defined state are committed to a given specific pathway. The basis of the dual action of FGF-1 has therefore been approached by using substances that interfere with the transducing pathways known to be activated by growth factors. Genistein and tyrphostin, two inhibitors of tyrosine kinases, inhibit both cell scattering and mitogenesis induced by FGF-1. Conversely, sodium orthovanadate, a potent inhibitor of tyrosine phosphatases, reproduces the two functions of FGF-1, indicating that protein tyrosine phosphorylation is an early determinant in the two pathways. However, there is evidence that the two pathways are divergent since TGF-β1 is a strong inhibitor of DNA synthesis induced by FGF-1 and yet has no effect on cell scattering. In an attempt to determine the specificity of the pathways of FGF-1, we found that the level of cAMP is of pivotal importance in distinguishing between the two transducing pathways leading to either

DNA replication or cell dispersion. Forskolin, 8-bromo cAMP, dibutyryl-cAMP and cholera toxin , which all increase cAMP levels, are all capable of potentiating the mitogenic effect of FGF-1, while strongly inhibiting its scattering action. Moreover, addition of any of these substances to converted, fibroblastic NBT-II cells immediately induces their reversion to an epithelial phenotype. These findings support a role for cAMP as a modulator of the effect of FGF-1 and in the establishment and maintenance of the epithelial state (Boyer and Thiery 1993).

The fact that the same growth factor can mediate two very different effects – cell scaterring at low cell density and cell proliferation at high density – suggest a very simple model for tumor development. At the center of the tumor, where the cell density of cells is high, the cells would proliferate, whereas at the edge of the tumors, the cells will scatter and migrate in the surrounding tissue. Collagens in the surrounding extracellular matrix synergize with certain growth factors to promote dissociation and locomotion of carcinoma cells, ultimately leading to metastasis to distant sites. We thus believe that the NBT-II in vitro model has helped us to define the conditions under which carcinomas progress to a more malignant phenotype.

8.1.3 Possible Involvement of src in the EMT of NBT-II Cells

One of our goals is to decipher the molecular mechanisms which lead either to cell dissociation or mitogenesis. Among the molecules known to be involved in the signaling pathways generated by growth factors, pp60c-src was particularly interesting because it has been shown to be involved in epithelial plasticity (Warren et al. 1988). We found that the pathway leading to EMT involves an early and sustained stimulation of pp60c-src kinase activity. This early activation was not observed during the mitogenic response. Several arguments suggest that pp60c-src is indeed involved in the EMT of NBT-II cells: (1) stable transfection of a dominant-negative mutant of c-src inhibits the scattering response without affecting mitogenesis induced by EGF or FGF-1; (2) overexpression of c-src causes a subpopulation of cells to undergo spontaneous EMT and sensitizes the rest of the population to the scattering activity of EGF and FGF-1, without affecting growth factor-induced mitogenesis (Rodier et al. 1995).

8.1.4 Effect of an Autocrine Production of FGF-1 by NBT-II Cells

We have generated FGF-1-producing NBT-II cells by transfection with recombinant expression vectors containing FGF-1 cDNA or the human FGF-1 cDNA coupled to a signal peptide sequence (SP-FGF-1; Jouanneau et al. 1991). The effects of both the nonsecreted and secreted human 16-kDa growth factor on morphology, motility, and cell invasiveness (gelatinase activity) have been compared. FGF-1 coupled to a signal peptide is actively secreted by the producing cells. The secretion of FGF-1 is not necessary for induction of gelatinase activity, as this has been observed in NBT-II cells producing FGF-1 with or without a signal peptide. Production of FGF-1 (whether secreted or not) results in an increase in cell motility of most isolated clones; however, there is no correlation between FGF-1 level and motility rate. These data suggest that expression of FGF-1 in NBT-II cells induces metastatic potential, through either an autocrine or intracrine mechanism.

To assay the effect of growth factors on cell invasiveness in a more complex and physiologically relevant model, we analyzed the behavior of NBT-II spheroids cocultured with urinary bladder in organotypic cultures (Tucker et al. 1991b). NBT-II spheroids progressively replaced the urothelium at the site of contact with the bladder explant. In the absence of growth factors, NBT-II cells grow in a pattern suggestive of local hyperplasia, with occasional cell protrusions. Exogenously added scatter/growth factors elicit a more rapid appearance of these protrusions, which are also more numerous. NBT-II cells transfected with FGF-1, TGF-α, or FGF-4 (hst/K-FGF) cDNA constructs were also used. TGF-α and FGF-4 can also induce EMT in NBT-II cells. After exogenous or autocrine stimulation of NBT-II cells with the growth/scatter factors, a deeper penetration of the bladder wall in the form of nodular outgrowths or clusters of infiltrating cells was always observed. These observations suggest that scatter/growth factors can promote cell shedding in NBT-II clusters and lead to an increase in invasiveness, even in the complex extracellular environment of bladder tissues.

8.2 A Community Effect for Tumor Progression

Tumor progression was also studied in vivo. In nude mice, growth factors can increase the tumorigenicity and the metastatic potential of NBT-II cells, the effect being particularly dramatic for FGF-1. We then addressed the question of whether cells that produce FGF-1 (or other scatter/growth factors) will behave within a tumor as a dominant cell population with a proliferative, invasive and/or metastatic advantage over the other cells, or whether they behave as nondominant variants, possibly functioning as helper cells in the primary tumor for cells which do not produce their own growth factors.

8.2.1 A Community Effect with NBT-II Cells Producing FGF-1

A minimum number of 3.5×10^6 NBT-II cells has to be injected subcutaneously in order to obtain a tumor. Tumors are never detected before 30 days. Tumor growth is rather slow since a 1000 mm^3 tumor is formed 2 months after injection. In sharp contrast, cells transfected with an FGF-1 cDNA without a signal peptide form a 1000 mm^3 tumor by day 10. Tumor size is similar for cells transfected with an FGF-1 cDNA construct containing a signal peptide; in the latter case, however, the tumor is more highly vascularized, reflecting the angiogenic effect of secreted FGF-1. Micrometastases are detected in lymph nodes within 12 days in the case of these very rapidly developing tumors. Micrometastases are also found with the untransfected NBT-II cells; these micrometastases appear later, perhaps as a consequence of the lag-time for the formation of the primary tumors.

We then asked whether FGF-1 producing cells within a carcinoma may be dominant for tumor proliferation and metastatic spreading. For that purpose we coinjected different mixtures of NBT-II cells and NBT-II cells transfected with FGF-1. These experiments mimic the heterogeneity of tumors, in which different clones of cancer cells often coexist. FGF-1 producing cells were mixed with control NBT-II cells in a ratio decreasing from 500 000 to 1000 transfected cells in a total of 3.5×10^6 cells. As few as three FGF-1-producing cells for 10 000 NBT-II cells can shorten by twofold the delay in the appearance of tumors and metastases. The tumor cells which grew in the primary tumors and in the metastases were a mixture of FGF-1-producing cells and normal NBT-II cells. The NBT-II cells could be recognized because they were transfected with the β-galactosidase gene. Apparently, FGF-1-producing cells are not dominant in vivo, but rather mediate a community effect within the tumor cell population, resulting in an increased tumorigenicity (Jouanneau et al. 1994).

8.2.2 The Community Effect Is Not Specific for FGF-1-Producing Cells

Factors other than FGF-1 may mediate a similar community effect in these cells. There is a spontaneous metastatic variant of the NBT-II cell line, M-NBT-II, which has been obtained by in vivo selection. This variant produces and secretes in the medium a factor which has epithelial cell-scattering activity. This factor, although sharing some properties with HGF/SF, has been partially characterized and is distinct from HGF (Bellusci et al. 1994b). M-NBT-II is much more tumorigenic than the parental cell line. The presence of M-NBT-II cells (14%) with NBT-II cells (86%) is sufficient to increase the tumorigenicity and subsequently the metastatic behavior of the entire cell population. Thus, as in the case of NBT-II cells transfected with FGF-1, there is no clonal dominance of the growth factor-producing cells for tumorigenicity and metastatic spreading, but rather a community effect (Bellusci et al. 1994–1995).

8.3 Concluding Remarks

These studies emphasize the role of multifunctional growth factors and their receptors in the progression of carcinoma. Most importantly it shows that a single growth factor can contribute to several different steps of tumor progression. It can promote the development of a primary tumor through its mitogenic and angiogenic properties. It can also promote local tumor invasion through its ability to induce the production of proteolytic activities and its scattering function. The community effect mediated by a subset of carcinoma cells producing a growth factor may be of the utmost importance in the development of heterogenous

162   F. Radvanyi et al.

tumors. Clones producing a growth factor may enhance the tumorigenic
and metastatic behavior of other clones. This novel finding raises questions about the possibility of identifying a limited number of genes
which would be considered as metastases promoting genes (metasto-
genes).

Work in progress in our laboratory is directed at the development of
in vivo models to assess the function of growth factors in the progression of carcinoma induced in situ by carcinogenic agents.

References

Bellusci S. Moens G, Baudino G, Comoglio P, Nakamura T, Thiery JP, Jouan-
    neau J (1994a) Creation of an hepatocyte growth factor/scatter factor
    autocrine loop in carcinoma cells induces invasive properties associated
    with increased tumorigenicity. Oncogene 9:1091–1099
Bellusci S, Moens G, Thiery JP, Jouanneau J (1994b) A scatter factor like fac-
    tor is produced by a metastatic variant of a rat bladder carcinoma cell line. J
    Cell Sci 107:1277–1287
Bellusci S, Moens G, Delouvee A, Thiery JP, Jouanneau J (1994–1995) SFL
    production by carcinoma cells induces the aggressive properties of nonpro-
    ducing cells in vivo via a community effect. Invas Met 14:319–328
Boyer B, Thiery JP (1993) Cyclic AMP distinguishes between two functions
    of acidic FGF in a rat bladder carcinoma cell line. J Cell Biol 120:767–776
Boyer B, Tucker GC, Vallés AM, Gavrilovic J, Thiery JP (1989a) Reversible
    transition towards a fibroblastic phenotype in a rat carcinoma cell line. Int J
    Cancer 4:69–75
Boyer B, Tucker GC, Vallés AM, Franke WW, Thiery JP (1989b) Rearrange-
    ments of desmosomal and cytoskeletal proteins during the transition from
    epithelial to fibroblastoid organization in cultured rat bladder carcinoma
    cells. J Cell Biol 109:1495–1509
Gavrilovic J, Moens G, Thiery JP, Jouanneau J (1990) Expression of trans-
    fected transforming growth factor alpha induces a motile fibroblast-like
    phenotype with extracellular matrix-degrading potential in a rat bladder car-
    cinoma cell line. Cell Regul 1:1003–1014
Jouanneau J, Gavrilovic J, Caruelle D, Jaye M, Moens G, Caruelle JP, Thiery
    JP (1991) Secreted or nonsecreted forms of acidic fibroblast growth factor
    produced by transfected epithelial cells influence cell morphology, motility,
    and invasive potential. Proc Natl Acad Sci USA 88:2893–2897

Jouanneau J, Moens G, Bourgeois Y, Poupon MF, Thiery JP (1994) A minority of carcinoma cells producing acidic fibroblast growth factor induces a community effect for tumor progression. Proc Natl Acad Sci USA 91:286–290

Matthay MA, Thiery JP, Lafont F, Stampfer F, Boyer B (1993) Transient effect of epidermal growth factor on the motility of an immortalized mammary epithelial cell line. J Cell Sci 106:869–878

Nakamura T, Nishizawa T, Hagiya M, Seki T, Shimonishi M, Sugimura A, Tashiro K, Shimizu S (1989) Molecular cloning and expression of human hepatocyte growth factor. Nature 342:440–443

Rodier JM, Vallés AM, Denoyelle M, Thiery JP, Boyer B (1995) pp60c-src is a positive regulator of growth factor-induced cell scattering in a rat bladder carcinoma cell line. J Cell Biol 131:761–773

Savagner P, Vallés AM, Jouanneau J, Yamada KM, Thiery JP (1994) Alternative splicing in fibroblast growth factor receptor 2 is associated with induced epithelial-mesenchymal transition in rat bladder carcinoma cells. Mol Biol Cell 5:851–862

Tchao R (1982) Novel forms of epithelial cell motility on collagen and on glass surfaces. Cell Motility 4:333–341

Toyoshima K, Ito N, Hiasa Y, Kamamoto Y, Makiura S (1971) Tissue culture of urinary bladder tumor induced in a rat by N-butyl-N-(4-hydroxybutyl)nitrosamine: establishment of cell line, Nara bladder tumor II. J Natl Cancer Inst 47:979–985

Tucker GC, Boyer B, Gavrilovic J, Emonard H, Thiery JP (1990) Collagen-mediated dispersion of NBT-II rat bladder carcinoma cells. Cancer Res 50:129–137

Tucker GC, Boyer B, Vallés AM, Thiery JP (1991a) Combined effects of extracellular matrix and growth factors on NBT-II rat bladder carcinoma cell dispersion. J Cell Sci 100:371–380

Tucker GC, Delouvee A, Jouanneau J, Gavrilovic J, Moens G, Vallés AM, Thiery JP (1991b) Amplification of invasiveness in organotypic cultures after NBT-II rat bladder carcinoma stimulation with in vitro scattering factors. Invasion Metastasis 11:297–309

Vallés AM, Boyer B, Badet J, Tucker GC, Barritault D, Thiery JP (1990a) Acidic fibroblast growth factor is a modulator of epithelial plasticity in a rat bladder carcinoma cell line. Proc Natl Acad Sci USA 87:1124–1128

Vallés AM, Tucker GC, Thiery JP, Boyer B (1990b) Alternative patterns of mitogenesis and cell scattering induced by acidic FGF as a function of cell density in a rat bladder carcinoma cell line. Cell Regul 1:975–988

Warren SL, Handel LM, Nelson WJ (1988) Elevated expression of pp60c-src alters a selective morphogenetic property of epithelial cells in vitro without a mitogenic effect. Mol Cell Biol 8:632–646

164   F. Radvanyi et al.

Weidner KM, Behrens J, Vandekerckhove J, Birchmeier W (1990) Scatter factor: molecular characteristics and effect on the invasiveness of epithelial cells. J Cell Biol 111:2097–2108

Weidner KM, Arakaki N, Hartmann G, Vandekerckhove J, Weingart S, Rieder H, Fonatsch C, Tsubouchi H, Hishida T, Daikuhara Y et al. (1991) Evidence for the identity of human scatter factor and human hepatocyte growth factor. Proc Natl Acad Sci USA 88:7001–7005

9 The Role of Epidermal Growth Factor Receptor in the Initiation and Progression of Malignancy

K. Khazaie

9.1 Introduction

Sequence homologies between the cellular platelet-derived growth factor (PDGF) and epidermal growth factor receptor (EGFR) with the products of retroviral simian sarcoma virus (SSV) v-sis (Doolittle et al. 1984; Waterfield et al. 1983) and avian erythroblastosis virus (AEV) v-erbB (Downward et al. 1984b) putative oncogenes provided strong support for the notion that deregulation of cellular growth control may form the basis for cancer. This was practically demonstrated in the case of avian erythroblastosis by functional replacement of v-erbB through human EGFR (Khazaie et al. 1988). Oncogenes and deregulation of cell proliferation provided a powerful tool for explaining cancer at the molecular level (Sinn et al. 1987).

However, the most life-threatening aspect of cancer is not the growth of a tumor by itself, but the progression of the tumor into disseminated and eventually lethal metastases that grow in multiple distant organs (Schirrmacher 1985). The link between tumor initiation, promotion, and progression is complex. In contrast to the extensive list of oncogenes and antioncogenes characterized in the past years, surprisingly few genes have been directly linked to malignant progression more precisely to the process of tumor metastasis (Günthert et al. 1991; Hart and Easty 1991; Leone et al. 1991). In addition, documented observations show correlations of gain or loss of different gene products during the progression of various cancers. The EGRF is one such notable example (Khazaie et al. 1993).

The molecular and cellular basis of metastasis is still the grayest area of cancer research and may be the most difficult one to solve mechanistically. Genomic instability and chaos in tumor cells and cell lines is at least in part responsible for the slow progress in defining these critical molecular events that push cancer cells into the metastatic phenotype. The work presented here covers three aspects of the carcinogenesis process:

1. Proliferation and survival of leukemia cells
2. Invasive growth of solid tumors
3. Tumor dissemination

Much of this work has focused on the EGFR, the first discovered growth factor receptor/protooncogene. Both in vitro assays and animal models were used to address questions of relevance to the lethality of malignancy, with a view to defining potential targets for therapy. Throughout, I have been motivated by the thought that a detailed knowledge of the nature of neoplasia will not only satisfy our sense of curiosity about the molecular and cellular basis of life but also provide us with opportunities for controlling cancer as a disease.

9.2 Role of EGFR in the Proliferation and Survival of Leukemia Cells: Constitutive Expression of the Epidermal Growth Factor Receptor Subverts Erythroid Differentiation and Causes Erythroleukemia in Chicks

9.2.1 Molecular Alterations of the v-erbB Oncogene

Cancer in birds is often caused by oncogenic retroviruses. These viruses have, through illegitimate recombination and gene transduction, exchanged part or all of their coding capacity with sequences encoding cDNA copies of cellular genes. Existence of such naturally occurring recombinant viruses became obvious in cases where expression of the ectopic genes in newly infected cells led to dysregulated growth and disease. Typical examples are avian leukemogenic viruses, which through multiple cyles of infection express defined oncogenes in a large population of hematopoietic cells, leading to polyclonal expansion of defined cell types and eventually to lethality.

The AEV is a classical member of the avian oncogenic retroviurses, causing an acute polyclonal erythroid leukemia and, depending on the isolate, fibrosarcoma. The ES4 strain of this virus was isolated through serial passage of a weak leukemia inducing virus (RAV1) in chicks (Engelbreth-Holm and Meyer 1935). It took no less than half a century to demonstrate the ability of this virus to expand erythroblasts and transform fibroblasts in vitro (Graf et al. 1976, 1977). Molecular cloning of the AEV-ES4 showed that the virus encoded two ectopic genes, v-erbA and v-erbB (Vennstrom et al. 1980; Fig. 1). Sequence homology

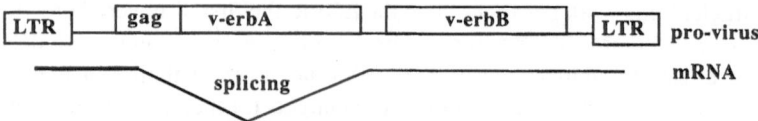

Fig. 1. Schematic representation of the avian erythroblastosis virus (AEV)-ES4 pro-virus and the transcribed mRNA. Note that v-erbA is expressed from a genomic, while the v-erbB from a subgenomic (spliced) transcript. *LTR*, long terminal repeat

to the human EGFR indicated that the v-erbB gene represents an altered version of the gene encoding the avian EGFR (Downward et al. 1984a,b). Similarly, the v-erbA oncogene was shown to correspond to an altered form of the thyroid hormone receptor (Sap et al. 1986). Detailed study of the molecular differences between the avian EGFR and the v-erbB oncogene has been instrumental in revealing the exact role of the transduced cellular gene in the expansion of chick erythroblasts and induction of fibrosarcoma.

In comparison with the complete human EGFR, the v-erbBES4 gene lacks 73 amino acids of the C-terminus and all except 70 amino acids of the ligand-binding domain (for review see Vennstrom et al. 1989). The ligand-binding domain exerts a negative regulatory effect on the tyrosine kinase activity of the EGFR, and removal of this region leads to constitutive receptor function (Khazaie et al. 1988). The missing C-terminal domain includes major tyrosine autophosphorylation sites of the EGFR. Phosphorylation of these tyrosine residues is important for the physical interaction of EGFR with other cellular proteins that carry compatible so-called src homology 2 (SH2) domains (see Fig. 1, and below). Furthermore, this domain appears to have a negative regulatory function, as truncation of the carboxy terminal domain has led to constitutive EGFR activity (Khazaie et al. 1988; Massoglia et al. 1990).

The SH2 domain is a common feature of many nonreceptor kinases which act in the signal cascade downstream of activated growth factor receptors. This is the major structural feature responsible for interaction of phospholiplase C-γ (PLC-γ), phosphatidyl inositol 3 (PI3) kinase, and ras-GTPase activating protein (GAP) with the activated EGFR. Recruitment of these molecules to the cell surface through "docking" with the autophosphorylated EGF C-terminal tyrosine residues and their subsequent phosphorylation and/or conformational modulation have been proposed to lead to their activation and secondary signal transduction. The affinity of EGFR for these molecules is variable, being high for PLC-γ but particularly low for PI3 kinase. Therefore, for some molecules and in some cell types successful interactions may dependent on the level of EGFR expression. Raf, a serine/threonine kinase which also associates with EGFR does not contain an SH2 domain. The complexities of such interactions have been used as a basis to explain the cooperation of different receptors in the activation of growth as well as transformation-associated changes (for reviews see: Khazaie et al. 1993). Nevertheless, receptor activation and function in intact cells surprisingly does not always seem to require tyrosine autophosphorylation and presumably exposure of these "docking" sites (Lichtner et al. 1992).

9.2.2 Structure and Function Relationship of EGFR to the Etiology of Erythroleukemia

To clarify the role of EGFR and the alterations observed in the v-erbB oncogene in eythroblastosis, molecular clones of the complete human EGFR (HER1) or truncated versions thereof (Fig. 2) were inserted into the AEV-ES4 virus, replacing the naturally occurring erbB oncogene (Khazaie et al. 1988).

Infectious recombinant virus particles were used to infect bone marrow explants in vitro or were injected into new born chicks. All constructs except those with 126 amino acid deletions of the carboxy terminal domain were able to expand chicken erythroblasts from the in vitro bone marrow cultures. Clearly, truncations of the carboxy or amino terminal ends of the EGFR removed dependence of the EGFR on presence of ligand. This result was supported by the ability of the truncated forms of the receptor to promote incorporation of [^{3}H]deoxythymidine in infected erythroblasts or fibroblasts in the absence of exogenous EGF. The leukemogenic potential of HER1 was confirmed by injection of the recombinant viruses into new-born chicks. In sensitive strains, the complete HER1 when combined with v-erbA could promote acute erythroblastosis. Truncation of HER1 allowed induction of erythroblastosis in relatively resistant chick strains. Thus, appropriate

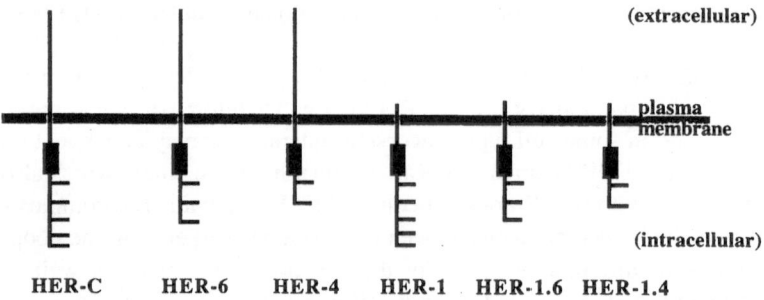

Fig. 2. Schematic representation of the complete full-length human epidermal growth factor receptor (*HER*) or truncated version thereof. Carboxy-terminal truncations removed 32 or 126 amino acids respectively. Amino terminal truncations removed all except for the signal peptide region of the extracellular domain. The major tyrosine autophosphorylation sites (amino acid positions 1186, 1173, 1148, 1086, 1068, and 992 respectively) on the carboxy terminal end of the receptor are represented as *small horizontal bars*, while the tyrosine kinase domain is shown by *dark boxes*

truncations of HER1 acted to remove dependence of HER1 on ligand, while v-erbA enhanced and complemented action of EGFR in erythroid transformation.

Shortly afterwards it was shown that immature erythroblasts, but not differentiated erythrocytes naturally express EGFR (Pain et al. 1991; Schroeder et al. 1993). Presumably, shut down of EGFR expression is a necessary event for terminal differentiation of erythroblasts since persistent expression of this receptor (even in an unmutated wild-type form) led to hyperproliferation of an immature polyclonal population of erythroid cells. Since the complete HER1 was shown to be leukemogenic, no particular change in structure/specificity of EGFR was needed for erythroblastosis. Nevertheless, truncation of the 32 C-terminal amino acids had a profound effect on the ability of the infected cells to survive spontaneous differentiation, in the absence of anemic serum (erythropoietin). Thus, a C-terminal truncation that removed the last two tyrosine autophosphorylation sites allowed erythropoietin-independent differentiation of erythroblasts to erythrocytes. This truncation changed the specificity of EGFR, allowing it to transmit signals normally characteristic of the erythropoietin receptor.

A further interesting insight into the structure/specificity relationship of the EGFR came from the finding that the 126 C-terminal truncation disabled erythroblast transformation, but enhanced fibroblast transformation. Thus, the amino acid residues immediately C-terminal to the tyrosine kinase domain are likely to be involved in interactions critical for EGFR-mediated erythroid (but not fibroblast) proliferation.

9.2.3 Aberrant Expression of EGFR Abrogates Dependence of Myeloid Leukemia Cells on Granulocyte Macrophage–Colony-Stimulating Factor, But Does Not Influence Myeloid Differentiation

Infection of chick bone marrow explants or of new born chicks with EGFR expressing retroviruses primarily induced erythroid expansions and erythroleukemia. This characteristic of EGFR was shared by nearly every other member of the cytoplasmic tyrosine kinase family of oncogenes. In contrast, the myeloid lineage appeared to be sensitive to transformation by nuclear oncogenes (for review see Beug and Graf 1989; Graf et al. 1988). Avian retroviruses MC29 and a particular substrain of MH2 are causative agents of chicken myelocytomatosis and monocytic leukemia (Graf and Beug 1978). The transforming activity of these viruses is due to their expression of v-myc (MC29) or a fusion product of the v-myc and the tyrosine kinase v-mil (avian homologue of v-raf) oncogenes (MH2). In contrast to MC29 transformed monocytes which were growth factor independent, in vitro expanded MH2 myeloid cells were strictly dependent on the presence of the chicken myelomonocytic growth factor (cMGF) (Leutz et al. 1984) for their survival and proliferation. It was postulated that EGFR may transmit survival functions compatible to those of cMGF or v-mil in v-myc transformed myeloid cells.

Thus, recombinant retroviral vectors were made that coexpressed the HER1 with v-myc oncogene of MC29 virus. Both genes were expressed from an AEV based vector (Fig. 3).

Indeed, v-myc transformed myeloid cells expressing the complete HER1 survived and proliferated in response to EGF instead of cMGF. The removal of 126 carboxy-terminal amino acids of HER1 (HER1-1.4) disabled this property of the receptor (Zenke et al. 1990). We had shown

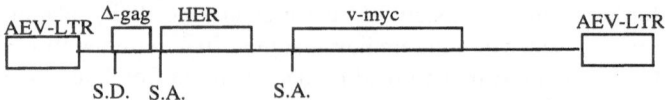

Fig. 3. Schematic representation of the retroviral vector used to express full-length human epidermal growth factor receptor (*HER*) and v-myc in chick bone marrow. *LTR*, long terminal repeats of avian erythroblastosis virus (*AEV*); S.D., splice donor site; S.A., splice acceptor site

earlier that the HER-1.4 mutant had no erythroblast transforming ability, while acting potently to transform fibroblasts. Thus it seems that the amino acid residues immediately carboxy-terminal to the tyrosine kinase domain of EGFR (residues 32—126 from the carboxy terminal end) have a critical function specific to hematopoietic cells.

Interestingly, coexpression of myc in murine IL-2 dependent hematopoietic cells was also shown to allow proliferation and survival of the cells in response to EGF (Shibuya et al. 1992). The myc product has been postulated to act as a transducing switch or filter for signals from EGFR and other tyrosine kinase growth factor receptor (Sorrentino et al. 1986). Indeed, the illegitimate cooperative action of myc and EGFR can disturb the proliferation of cells of a variety of differentiation lineages across the species, promoting neoplastic growth.

9.3 Role of EGFR in the Invasive Growth of Solid Tumors

9.3.1 Action of EGFR Is Critical for the Sarcomagenic Growth of myc Transformed Fibroblasts

The close sequence homology of HER1 and the v-erbB, a sarcomagenic oncogene, as well as the overexpression of HER1 in the A431 human carcinoma cell line suggested a possible role for EGFR in the malignant transformation of fibroblasts and epithelial cells (Downward et al. 1984b; Ullrich et al. 1984). Since both of these cell types normally express EGFR, the question was whether overexpression of EGFR was sufficient for tumorigenic growth. To test this, AEV-based retroviral vectors expressing HER1 alone or in combination with v-myc or v-erbA

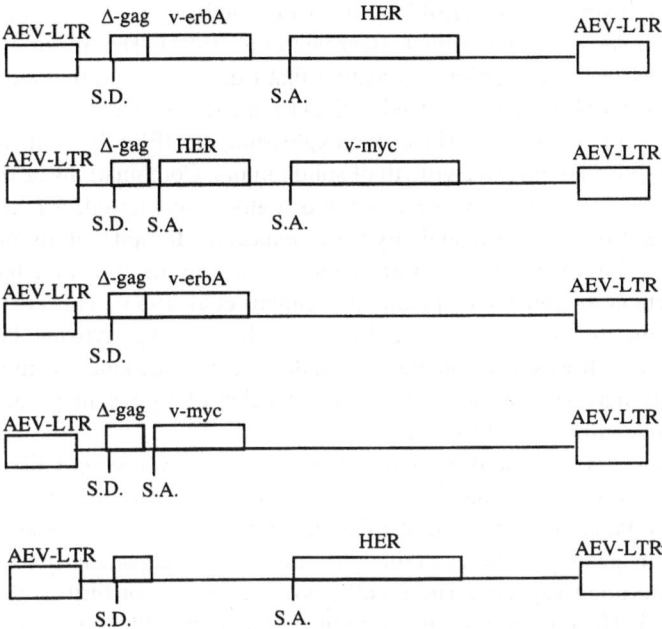

Fig. 4. Schematic representation of the retroviral vector used to express full-length human epidermal growth factor receptor (*HER*), v-myc or v-erbA or combinations of these in chick embryo fibroblasts. *LTR,* long terminal repeats of avian erythroblastosis virus (*AEV*); S.D., splice donor site; S.A., splice acceptor site

were used to infect chicken embryo fibroblasts (CEFs; Fig. 4). As control, similar vectors expressing v-myc or v-erbA alone were used.

The genetically altered fibroblasts were tested for their tumorigenic growth on the chorioallantoic membrane (CAM) of embryonated chick eggs. The CAM provides an easily accessible and immunologically defficient living membrane. Thus, it allows analysis of tumorigenic properties of cells, avoiding complications that may arise from an anti-tumor immune response. Murine NIH-3T3 cells were transfected with an expression vector encoding EGF and tested for secretion of EGF. These were irradiated and coinjected with CEFs genetically modified to express HER1, or nuclear oncogenes, or combinations of these.

Overexpression of HER1 by itself or together with v-erbA did not lead to sarcomagenic growth (Khazaie et al. 1991). This result agreed with earlier investigations indicating that truncations and mutations of the chick EGFR may be indeed critical for the sarcomagenic potential of the v-erbB oncogene. Thus, overexpression of HER1 is unlikely by itself to lead to invasive growth of solid tumors. Combinations of HER1 and other nuclear oncogenes, v-myb or v-myc, were tested. A potential cooperation of EGFR and myc was expected. In spite of its potent stimulation of fibroblast proliferation in vitro, by itself, v-myc has no detectable sarcomagenic potential (Palmieri et al. 1983). This contrasts with the sarcomagenic potential of v-src, the prototype tyrosine kinase oncogene. It was therefore postulated that the tyrosine kinase activity of EGFR may compensate for the deficiencies of v-myc in promoting invasive growth of fibroblasts.

Indeed, paracrine provision of EGF to v-myc expressing CEFs produced vascularized and invasive tumors on the CAM (Khazaie et al. 1991). Paracrine provision of EGF and expression of v-myb also led to sarcomagenic growth, even though v-myb has no apparaent fibroblast-transforming capacity. These cells, however, were not further characterized. The rate-limiting function of EGF is highly likely to be related to changes in contact and communication of the cells with their microenvironment (La Rocca et al. 1989). EGFR is a known stimulant of cellular proteolytic enzymes as well as a potent motility factor (for review see Khazaie et al. 1993).

9.4 Role of EGFR in Tumor Dissemination

9.4.1 EGFR Promotes Metastasis
of Mammary Adenocarcinoma Cells

Analysis of clinical data indicates that expression of the EGFR could play an important role in tumor progression. The amplification of the EGFR (c-erbB) locus has been associated with the progression of several human tumors of epidermal and glial origin. In human breast tumors a strong inverse correlation between the expression of estrogen receptor and EGFR has been established. High expression of EGFR has been considered to account for a poor prognosis in breast carcinoma patients, and expression of the receptor is reported to be elevated in breast tumor metastases as compared to the primary tumor. However, a causative link between expression of EGFR and the process of metastasis has been difficult to established (for review see Khazaie et al. 1993).

We exploited a well-defined rat mammary tumor model to demonstrate a role for EGFR in metastasis. An earlier report had documented differential response to EGF of two closely related epithelial cell tumor clones with equal tumorigenic but contrasting metastatic potential isolated from the 13762NF rat mammary adenocarcinoma (Neri et al. 1982). Only the highly metastatic clone MTLn3 responded in vitro to EGF with an increase in cell proliferation, while the nonmetastatic clone MTC was not affected (Lichtner et al. 1988). The two cell lines were investigated in detail for expression and function of EGFR. To test the role of EGFR in metastasis, an ectopic human EGFR was expressed in the low metastatic cell line; the genetically modified cells were cloned and subjected to extensive analyses.

9.4.2 Expression of EGFR Correlates with Metastatic Potential of Rat Mammary Adenocarcinoma Cells

Analysis of EGFR transcripts in the rat mammary carcinoma cell lines suggested that the EGFR locus in these cells was not productively rearranged, leading, for example, to v-erbB like truncations of the rat EGFR (Lichtner et al. 1992). Cross-linking experiments with ^{125}I-labeled EGF, as well as [^{35}S]methionine labelling followed by immunoprecipitation with receptor-specific antibodies readily detected in MTLn3 cells the expected 170-kDa EGFR protein. In addition, two proteins with M_r of 420—480 and 95 kDa specifically bound ^{125}I-labeled EGF on intact MTLn3 cells. In agreement with the reported structure and properties of the secretory form of EGFR molecule, the 95-kDa molecule derived from MTLn3 cells was not recognized by antibodies raised against the intracellular domain of EGFR and were not phosphorylated under any of the assay conditions used.

Detailed characterization of the high metastatic EGF-responsive clone MTLn3 revealed 1.0×10^4 high and 4.6×10^4 low- and high-affinity cell surface EGFR molecules. Surprisingly, while EGF-dependent phosphorylation of substrates occurred in intact cells, no receptor phosphorylation could be identified in intact cells or in membrane preparations. Indications for active suppression of receptor phosphorylation came from the fact that detergent stripping of membrane components unmasked this activity (Lichtner et al. 1992).

The extent to which these novel properties of MTLn3 may relate to their metastatic property is difficult to establish. Yet, an easy to test postulate was made based on the dramatic difference in expression of EGFR in the low metastatic MTC cells. The MTC cells exhibited low to undetectable levels of EGFR expression. Both cell lines however expressed transforming growth factor-α (TGF-α), a specific ligand to EGFR (Kaufmann et al. 1994). Thus, the possibility for an autocrine loop in MTLn3 was raised. The MTC cells were presumably spared from this autocrine loop since they did not express the receptor.

9.4.3 Expression of Ectopic EGFR Promotes Lung Colonization of Rat Mammary Adenocarcinoma Cells

In order to test for a causal role of EGFR in events associated with the metastatic process, a full-length cDNA to the normal human EGFR was introduced and expressed in MTC cells by means of a replication defective MoMLV based retroviral vector (Fig. 5). As control, the vector without human EGFR cDNA was used to generate G418 resistant control cells (MTC neo).

A combination of Northern blot analysis, immunoprecipitation with EGFR specific antibodies, and Scatchard analysis was used to demonstrate expression of the intact human EGFR. The expected transcripts and 170-kDa protein representing the human EGFR could be identified in MTC-HER1 cells. The ligand-binding properties of the human EGFR expressed on transfected cells was studied with ^{125}I-labeled EGF. While no binding was seen with MTC or MTC neo cells, MTC HER1 cells bound ^{125}I-labeled EGF. Scatchard analysis indicated that the human EGFR was expressed in MTC HER1 cells at levels comparable to the endogenous rat EGFR in MTLn3 cells and that it was capable of binding EGF with the expected affinities. The frequency of cells expressing HER1 was investigated with fluorescence-activated cell sorter (FACS) analysis, and FACS sorting was used to isolate clones of MTC-HER1 that stably and uniformly expressed the HER1 (S+). The independence

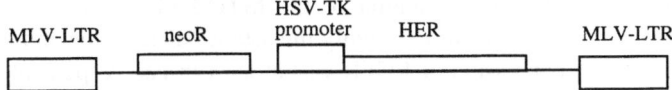

Fig. 5. Schematic representation of the retroviral vector used to express full-length human epidermal growth factor receptor (*HER*) in rat mammary carcinoma cells. *neoR,* neomycin resistance gene; *LTR,* long terminal repeats of Moloney leukemia virus (*MLV*)

of the clones was confirmed by Southern analysis, and the stability of the clones was checked by extensive in vitro passage, followed by FACS analysis for expression of EGFR.

It remained to be shown that the human receptor was functionally active in the transfected rat tumor cells. Receptor kinase activity of HER1 in transfected cells was demonstrated in immune precipitates of HER1 from extracts of MTC-HER1 cells. In contrast to the lack of receptor autophosphorylation in MTLn3 cells, ligand-dependent HER1 autophosphorylation was detectable in intact MTC-HER1 cells. Both MTLn3 and MTC-HER1 cells responded to EGF by exhibiting enhanced rates of adhesion to fibronectin or collagen in vitro (Lichtner et al. 1995).

When injected intravenously into female nude mice, the MTC-HER1 population was six- to sevenfold more metastatic than the parental untransfected cells, but only twofold more metastatic than the neoR control. Pretreatment of the MTC-HER1 or S+ clones but not MTC or MTCneo cells with EGF led to increase in lung-colonizing potential. These results were confirmed by experiments in which a pool of seven independent transfectants stably expressing HER1 was used. The number of lung colonies was now at least four times higher than MTC-neo control cells and increased significantly by pretreatment of the cells with EGF. Two individual S+ clones also showed a clear response to pretreatment with EGF, exhibiting enhanced lung-colonizing potential by 37- or threefold, respectively. The metastatic lung nodules showed prominent expression of HER1, as revealed by staining of isolated cells with anti-EGFR antibody, followed by fluorescence microscopy (Lichtner et al. 1995).

The lung-colonizing potential of the MTC-HER1 and S+ clones resembled the behavior of the highly metastatic MTLn3 line and demonstrated that expression of EGFR was at least in part responsible for the contrasting metastatic behavior of the two parental lines, MTC and MTLn3.

9.4.4 EGFR Promotes Spontaneous Metastasis of Rat Mammary Adenocarcinoma Cells, While Transmitting Antiproliferative Signals

Exogenous recombinant TGF-α significantly reduced the rate of proliferation of pools of S+ cells, as measured by the incorporation of [^{3}H]thymidine. Control MTC parental cells, which were devoid of EGFR, did not respond to TGF-α. In agreement with the proliferation analysis, ligand-specific stimulation of HER1 led to enhanced cell death in the pool of S+ cells, evidenced by the uptake of propidium iodide by unfixed cells. As expected EGF or TGF-α did not affect the survival of MTC cells. A minimum of 3 days continuous exposure to TGF-α was required for loss of cell viability.

The antiproliferative effects of TGF-α were related to degradation and release of genomic DNA, a hallmark of apoptosis. Significant loss of DNA in a TGF-α stimulated pool of S+ clones was detected already 2 days after exposure to TGF-α. In contrast, MTC cells showed no growth factor-dependent DNA loss. The loss of nuclear DNA by S+ cells correlated with a decrease in the proportion of cells in cycle, while the parental MTC cells were not affected. Morphological signs of apoptosis were detectable after a 3- to 4-day incubation of S+ cells with exogenous TGF-α. These morphological changes were blocked by inclusion in the culture medium of the ICR16 monoclonal anti-HER1 antibody, which specifically blocks interaction of ligand with HER1.

The antiproliferative effect of HER1 expression observed in vitro was also reflected in the behavior of S+ cells after orthotopic implantation (into the mammary fat pad) in nu/nu mice. Upon inoculation, both the uncloned MTC-HER1 cells and control MTC-neo cells grew more slowly than parental MTC. To check for apoptosis of tumor cells in situ, the frequency of double-strand breaks in intact cells was quantitated by an in situ terminal transferase assay. In agreement with earlier results,

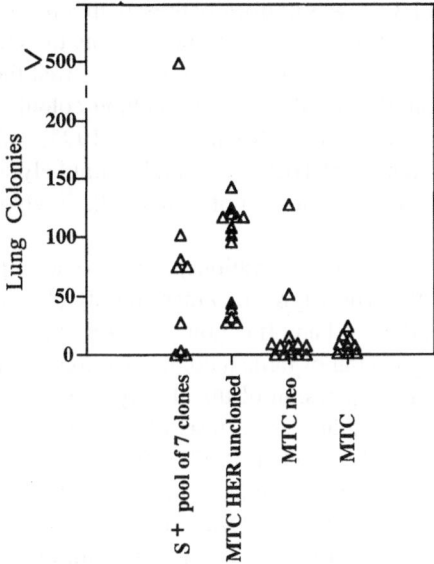

Fig. 6. Spontaneous metastasis of MTC cells modified to express full length human epidermal growth factor receptor

the pool of S+ cells cultured in the presence of TGF-α showed significantly higher numbers of apoptotic cells than untreated S+ cells. Similar results were seen in sections of primary tumor tissues that were subjected to terminal transferase reaction. Significantly higher levels of double-strand breaks in genomic DNA of S+ tumor cells were detected, in comparison to the parental MTC or control MTC-neo cells. Presumably an autocrine loop was engaged, stimulating the cell surface-expressed HER1 in vivo. This loop was presumably less important when the cells were sparsely cultured in vitro, allowing detection of response to exogenously added growth factor. These observations corroborated the in vitro data showing that HER1 promoted apoptotic death of S+ cells in vitro as well as in vivo.

In spite of the growth and survival disadvantages which resulted from the expression of HER1, S+ clones inoculated into the mammary fat pad were significantly more metastatic than the parental MTC or MTC-neo cells (Fig. 6).

Expression of HER1 was uniformly present in tumors and metastases derived from inoculation of S+ clones, underlining the stability of HER1 expression in the selected clones. The data supported the earlier report of EGF-dependent, enhanced adhesion and lung-colonizing potential of intravenously injected S+ cells (Lichtner et al. 1995) and indicated that the metastatic potential of HER1 was highly unlikely to be related to enhanced proliferation or survival of tumor cells in vivo (Kaufmann et al. 1996).

In addition to our own observations, several other reports have suggested a role for the type 1 tyrosine kinase family of receptors in tumor metastasis. Thus, the level and function of EGFR expression was linked to the metastatic potential of human colon carcinoma cells (Radinsky et al. 1995). Similarly, expression of the closely related c-erB2/neu oncogene was reported to induce metastasis of murine 3T3 fibroblasts and human lung cancer cells (Yu et al. 1992, 1994). Signal transduction from cell surface growth factor receptors can influence a wide range of events, including enhanced proliferation (Ozawa et al. 1987) or survival (Englert et al. 1995; Merlo et al. 1995), and it is often difficult to distinguish a direct influence of such receptors on tumor dissemination from indirect effects. Our observations clearly distinguished between the metastatic and growth/survival functions of EGFR (Kaufmann et al. 1996).

References

Beug H, Graf T (1989) Co-operation between viral oncogenes in avian erythroid and myeloid leukaemia. Eur J Clin Invest 19:491–502

Doolittle RF, Hunkapiller MW, Hood LE, Devare SG, Robbins KC, Aaronson SA, Antoniadis HN (1984) Simian sarcoma virus onc gne, v-sis, is derived from the gene (or genes) encoding a platelet-derived growth factor. Science 221:275–277

Downward J, Parker P, Waterfield MD (1984a) Autophosphorylation sites on the epidermal growth factor receptor. Nature 311:483–485

Downward J, Yarden Y, Mayes E, Scrace G, Totty N, Stockwell P, Ullrich A, Schlessinger J, Waterfield MD (1984b) Close similarity of epidermal growth factor receptor and v-erb-B oncogene protein sequences. Nature 307:521–527

Engelbreth-Holm J, Meyer AR (1935) Acta Pathol Microbiol Scand 12:352–365

Englert C, Hou X, Maheswaran S, Bennett P, Ngwu C, Re GG, Garvin AJ, Rosner MR, Haber DA (1995) WT1 suppresses synthesis of the epidermal growth factor receptor and induces apoptosis. EMBO J 14:4662–4675

Graf T, Beug H (1978) Avian leukemia viruses, interaction with their target cells in vivo and in vitro. Biochim Biophys Acta 516:269–299

Graf T, Royer PB, Schubert GE, Beug H (1976) Evidence for the multiple on-cogenic potential of cloned leukemia virus: in vitro and in vitro studies with avian erythroblastosis virus. Virology 71:423–433

Graf T, Fink D, Beug H, Royer PB (1977) Oncornavirus-induced sarcoma for-mation obscured by rapid development of lethal leukemia. Cancer Res 37:59–63

Graf T, Kahn P, Leutz A, Beug H, Vennstrom B (1988) Cooperativity of viral oncogenes in avian leukaemia. IARC Sci Publ *165–170

Günthert U, Hofmann M, Rudy W, Reber S, Zoller M, Haussmann I, Matzku S, Wenzel A, Ponta H, Herrlich P (1991) A new variant of glycoprotein CD44 confers metastatic potential to rat carcinoma cells. Cell 65:13–24

Hart IR, Easty D (1991) Identification of genes controlling metastatic behav-iour [editorial] [see comments]. Br J Cancer 63:9–12

Kaufmann A, Khazaie K, Kittmann A, Wiedemuth M, Illrich A, Schirrmacher V, Lichtner R (1994) Expression of EGF receptor correlates with metastatic potential of 13762 rat mammary adenocarcinoma. Int J Oncol 4:1149–1155

Kaufmann A, Lichtner R A, Schirrmacher V, Khazaie K (1996) Induction of apoptosis by EGF receptor in rat mammary adenocarcinoma cells coincides with enhanced tumour metastasis. (submitted)

Khazaie K, Dull TJ, Graf T, Schlessinger J, Ullrich A, Beug H, Vennstrom B (1988) Truncation of the human EGF receptor leads to differential trans-forming potentials in primary avian fibroblasts and erythroblasts. Embo J 7:3061–3071

Khazaie K, Panayotou G, Aguzi A, Samarut J, Gazzolo L, Jurdic P (1991) EGF promotes in vivo growth of primary checke embryo fibroblasts ex-pressing v-myc and enhances in vitro transformation by the v-erbA onco-gene. Oncogene 6:21–28

Khazaie K, Schirrmacher V, Lichtner RB (1993) EGF receptor in neoplasia and metastasis. Cancer Metastasis Rev 12:255–274

La Rocca S, Grossi M, Falcone G, Alema S, Tato F (1989) Interaction with normal cells suppresses the transformed phenotype of v-myc-transformed quail muscle cells. Cell 58:123–31

Leone A, Flatow U, King CR, Sandeen MA, Margulies IMK, Liotta LA, Steeg PS (1991) Reduced tumor incidence, metastatic potential, and cytokine re-sponsiveness of nm23-transfected melanoma cells. Cell 65:25–35

Leutz A, Beug H, Graf T (1984) Purification and characterization of cMGF, a novel chicken myelomonocytic growth factor. EMBO J 3:3191–7

Lichtner R, Gallick GE, Nicoslon GL (1988) Pyrimido-pyrimidine modulation of EGF growth-promoting activity and p21 ras expression in rat mammary adenocarcinoma cells. J Cell Physiol 137:285–292

Lichtner RB, Wiedemuth M, Kittmann A, Ullrich A, Schirrmacher V, Khazaie K (1992) Ligand-induced activation of EGFR in intact rat mammary adenocarcinoma cells without detectable receptor phosphorylation. J Biol Chem 267:11872–11880

Lichtner RB, Kaufmann AM, Kittmann A, Rohde SB, Walter J, Williams L, Ullrich A, Schirrmacher V, Khazaie K (1995) Ligand mediated activation of ectopic EGF receptor promotes matrix protein adhesion and lung colonization of rat mammary adenocarcinoma cells. Oncogene 10:1823–32

Massoglia S, Gray A, Dull TJ, Munemitsu S, Kung H-J, Schlessinger J, Ullrich A (1990) Epidermal growth factor receptor cytoplasmic domain mutations trigger ligand-independent transformation. Mol Cell Biol 10:3048–3055

Merlo GR, Basolo F, Fiore L, Laetitia D, Hynes NE (1995) p53-dependent and p53-independent activation of apoptosis in mammary epithelial cells reveals a survival function of EGF and insulin. J Cell Biol 128:1185–1196

Neri A, Welch D, Kawaguchi T, Nicolson GL (1982) Development and biologic properties of malignant cell sublines and clones of a spontaneously metastasizing rat mammary adenocarcinoma. J Natl Cancer Inst 68:507–517

Ozawa S, Ueda M, Ando N, Abe O, Hirai M, Shimizu N (1987) Stimulation by EGF of the growth of EGF receptor-hyperproducing tumor cells in athymic mice. Int J Cancer 40:706–710

Pain B, Woods CM, Saez J, Flickinger T, Raines M, Peyrol S, Moscovici C, Moscovici MG, Kung H-J, Jurdic P, Lazarides E, Samarut J (1991) EGF-R as a hemopoietic growth factor receptor: the c-erbB product is present in chicken erythrocytic progenitors and controls their self-renewal. Cell 65:37–46

Palmieri S, Kahn P, Graf T (1983) Quail embryo fibroblasts transformed by four v-myc containing virus isolates show enhanced proliferation but are non tumorigenic. EMBO J 2:2385–2389

Radinsky R, Seymon R, Fan D, Dong Z, Bielenberg D, Bucana CD, Fidler IJ (1995) Level and function of epidermal growth factor receptor predicts the metastatic potential of human colon carcinoma cells. Clin Cancer Res 1:19–31

Sap J, Munoz A, Damm K, Goldberg Y, Ghysdael J, Leutz A, Beug H, Vennstrsm B (1986) The c-erb-A protein is a high affinity receptor for thyroid hormone. Nature 324:635–640

Schirrmacher V (1985) Cancer metastasis: experimental approaches, theoretical concepts, and impacts for treatment strategies. Adv Cancer Res 43:1–73

Schroeder C, Gibson L, Nordström C, Beug H (1993) The estrogen receptor cooperates with the TGFα receptor (c-erbB) in regulation of chicken erythroid progenitor self-renewal. EMBO J 12:951–960

Shibuya H, Yoneyama M, Ninomiya TJ, Matsumoto K, Taniguchi T (1992) IL-2 and EGF receptors stimulate the hematopoietic cell cycle via different signaling pathways: demonstration of a novel role for c-myc. Cell 70:57–67

Sinn E, Muller W, Pattengale P, Tepler I, Wallace R, Leder P (1987) Co-expression of MMTV/v-Ha-ras and MMTVc-myc genes in transgenic mice: synergistic action of oncogenes in vivo. Cell 49:465–475

Sorrentino V, Drozdoff V, Mckinney MD, Zeitz L, Fleissner E (1986) Potentiation of growth factor activity by exogenous c-myc expression. Proc Natl Acad Sci USA 83:8167–8171

Ullrich A, Coussens L, Hayflick JS, Dull TJ, Gray A, Tam AW, Lee J, Yarden Y, Libermann TA, Schlessinger J, Downward J, Mayes ELV, Whittle N, Waterfield MD, Seeburg PH (1984) Human epidermal growth factor receptor cDNA sequence and aberrant expression of the amplified genes in A431 epidermoid carcinoma cells. Nature 309:418–425

Vennstrom B, Fanshier L, Moscovici C, Bishop JM (1980) Molecular cloning of the avian erythroblastosis virus genome and recovery of oncogenic virus by transfection of chicken cells. J Virol 36:575–85

Vennstrom B, Beug H, Forest D, Johnsson A, Khazaie K, Munoz A, Sap J, Ullrich A, Zenke M (1989) Functions of the erbA and erbB oncogenes in avian erythroblastosis. In: de Laat SW, Bluemink JG, Mummery CL (eds) Proceedings of the NATO advanced research workshop on cell to cell signalling in mammalian development. Springer, Berlin Heidelberg New York (NATO ASI Series, vol H26)

Waterfield MD, Scarce GT, Whittle N, Stroobant P, Johnsson A, Wasteson A, Westermark B, Heldin CH, Huang JS, Deuel TF (1983) Platelet-derived growth factor is structurally related to the putative transforming protein p28sis of simian sarcoma virus. Nature 304:35–39

Yu D, Hamada J, Zhang H, Nicolson GL, Hung MC (1992) Mechanism of c-erbB2/neu oncogene-induced metastasis and repression of metastatic properties by adenovirus 5 E1A gene products. Oncogene 7:2263–2271

Yu D, Wang SS, Dulski KM, Tsai CM, Nicolson GL, Hung MC (1994) c-erbB2/neu overexpression enhances metastatic potential of human lung cancer cells by induction of metastasis-associated properties. Cancer Res 54:3260–3266

Zenke M, Khazaie K, Beug H (1990) V-myc transformed macrophages expressing the normal human EGF receptor are induced to proliferate by EGF via a nonautocrine mechanism. In: Sachs L, Abraham NG, Wiedermann CJ, Levine AS, Konwalinka G (eds)Molecular biology of hematopoiesis. Intercept, Andover

10 Preclinical Studies with Human Tumour Xenografts Using Rat Monoclonal Antibodies Directed Against the Epidermal Growth Factor Receptor

S.A. Eccles, H. Modjtahedi, W. Court, J. Titley, G. Box, and C. Dean

10.1 Introduction

There is abundant evidence to suggest that over-expression of growth factor receptors and/or autocrine production of one or more ligands may provide tumour cells with significant advantages in growth and dissemination. One clinically important group is that of the c-erbB family of type 1 receptor tyrosine kinases exemplified by epidermal growth factor receptor (EGFR; reviewed by Harris et al. 1992; Khazaie et al. 1993; Modjtahedi and Dean 1994; Baselga and Mendelsohn 1994; Eccles et al. 1995). The cell surface location of these molecules renders them attractive targets for a variety of immunotherapeutic strategies, some of which are showing promise in preclinical and early clinical trials.

A number of murine monoclonal antibodies (mabs) directed primarily against the human EGFR receptor on the vulval carcinoma A431 have been described, some of which were shown to be growth inhibitory to EGFR over-expressing tumours in vitro and/or in vivo (reviewed in Modjtahedi and Dean 1994). We have generated a panel of rat mabs (which are generally of higher affinity and stability) against the EGFR expressed on a variety of different tumour cells for the following reasons: in A431 cells the gene is rearranged, the cells secrete an aberrant truncated form of the receptor, and many of the murine mabs produced crossreact with carbohydrate determinants on the blood group A antigen (Sato et al. 1987). We hoped that this strategy would yield a diverse population of mabs (in terms of epitope recognition and isotype) from which the best mab or combination of mabs could be selected for clinical development. This paper summarises our preclinical evaluation of a number of these mabs and our findings regarding potential mechanisms of action.

10.2 Materials and Methods

10.2.1 Monoclonal Antibodies

Rat monoclonal antibodies (mabs) recognising the external domain of the human EGFR were produced by immunising animals with live human tumour cell lines. A summary of their characteristics is listed in Table 1. Four different tumour types have been employed as immuno-

Table 1. Selected ICR monoclonal antibodies against external domains of human epidermal growth factor receptor

Mab	Immunogen	Epitope	Isotype	IC50 (nM)	Affinity (nM)	Reference
ICR9*	HN5	A	γ2a	*Promotes	3.5	Modjtahedi et al. 1993a,b
ICR10	HN5	B	γ2a	7.2	6.7	
ICR11	HN5	C	γ2a	0.8	5.0; 1.2	
ICR16*	HN5	C	γ2a	0.5	0.37; 3.7	
ICR61*	MDA MB 468	D	γ2b	8.7	0.25; 1.4	Modjtahedi et al. 1993c,d
ICR62*	MDA MB 468	C	γ2b	2.4	7.5	
ICR63	MDA MB 468	C	γ2a	2.8	0.15	
ICR64*	MDA MB 468	D	γ1	0.9	0.61; 1.8	
ICR65	MDA MB 468	C/D	γ2b	7.2	nd	
ICR76	A431	B	γ2a	>10	nd	Modjtahedi and Dean 1994
ICR78	A431	B	γ2a	>10	nd	
ICR79	A431	A/B	γ1	>10	nd	
ICR80	A172	D	γ1	2.1	nd	Modjtahedi et al. 1995b

nd, Not determined.

gens: HN5 squamous cell carcinoma (Modjtahedi et al. 1993b), MDA MB 468 breast carcinoma (Modjtahedi et al. 1993c), A431 vulval epidermoid carcinoma (Modjtahedi and Dean 1994) and A172 glioblastoma (Modjtahedi et al. 1995). Antibodies were purified from ascitic fluid as previously described (Modjtahedi et al. 1993b). Isotype matched control antibodies were used as controls, namely ALN/11/53 (IgG2a) and 11/160 (IgG2b) which recognise a specific antigen (NG2) on the rat chondrosarcoma HSN and RC1/4/74 (IgG1), an antibody directed against an idiotypic determinant on mab ICR16.

Table 2. Human tumour cell lines used in preclinical Mab testing

Cell line	Tumour type	No. EGFR	Ligand secretion
HN5	Squamous carcinoma	1.4×10^7	nd
A431	Squamous carcinoma	2.6×10^6	TGF-α; truncated EGFR
MDA MB 468	Breast carcinoma	1.5×10^6	TGF-α; (IGF1+ R)
SKOV 3	Ovarian carcinoma	$<10^5$	nd
A549	Lung adenocarcinoma	5×10^4 (+)	TGF-α; NDF
A172	Glioblastoma	$<10^4$	TGF-α

EGFR, epidermal growth factor receptor; TGF-α, transforming growth factor; IGF, insulin-like growth factor; NDF, neu differentiation factor; nd, not determined.

10.2.2 Tumour Cell Lines and Xenografts

The following human tumour cell lines were maintained in vitro in Dulbecco's modified Eagle's medium (DMEM) plus 10% heat inactivated foetal calf serum (FCS): A431, MDA MB 468, LICR-LON-HN5, A172, (described above) plus SKOV3 ovarian carcinoma and A549 lung adenocarcinoma. Their properties are summarised in Table 2. To assess the effect of mabs on the growth of human tumour xenografts, two basic treatment schedules were used.

10.2.2.1 Mab Treatment at the Time of Tumour Cell Inoculation
Five million tumour cells released from tissue culture flasks using trypsin-ethylene diamine tetraacetate (EDTA) were inoculated bilaterally s.c. in the flanks of 4- to 5-week-old female nu/nu mice in 100µl phosphate-buffered saline (PBS). On day 0, groups of four to six mice were dosed with 200µg of anti-EGFR mab and further groups received equal amounts of isotype-matched control mab or saline when previous experiments had shown no significant effects. Treatment was continued for a further 4 consecutive days and then thrice weekly, usually until 11 doses (total 2.2 mg) of mabs had been delivered. In some experiments, treatment was terminated earlier if complete eradication of tumour was observed, and in others lower doses were employed as outlined in the Sect. 10.3. Tumours were regularly measured across two perpendicular diameters (d1 and d2) and their volumes (V -expressed as cm^3) calculated from the formula: V=4/3[(d1+d2)4]3. Mice were killed when their

tumours reached a mean diameter of 0.8–1.0 cm, when the tumours were excised and weighed. If tumours regressed partially or completely, the mice were observed for up to 100 days when the experiment was terminated.

For comparison between groups where therapeutic responses resulted in different periods of growth, or for comparisons between different experiments, an average growth rate (GR) was calculated for each tumour. GR (mg/day)=weight of tumour at excision/growth period in days. Where tumours had regressed completely, GR was taken as 0.

10.2.2.2 Mab Treatment of Established Tumours

Xenograft tumours were initiated as before, but treatment was delayed until tumours had reached a mean diameter of 0.5 cm (mean volume 0.075 cm^3). Unless otherwise stated, mab treatment was as before; five consecutive daily doses with 200μg followed by thrice weekly dosing up to a total of 2.2 mg.

10.2.3 Histological Examination of Tumour Xenografts

At termination of experiments, tumours were fixed in modified Methacarn, paraffin embedded, sectioned at 4μm and stained with H&E for histological examination. In some cases, tumours were removed at earlier time points, cryopreserved and stained using peroxidase-conjugated F(ab')$_2$ rabbit anti-rat antibody to determine the localisation of therapeutic antibody (Modjtahedi et al. 1994).

10.2.4 Relative Expression of EGFR on Tumour Cells Determined by Fluorescence-Activated Cell Sorter

Cells were released from culture flasks using trypsin EDTA and incubated on a roller for 1 h at 4°C with saturating concentrations (10μg/ml) of rat anti-EGFR mab ICR62 in DMEM plus 10% FCS. Excess mab was removed by three washes with ice-cold PBS, and the cells were then incubated with fluorescein isothiocyanate (FITC)-conjugated sheep-anti rat Ig for a futher 1 h as before. Following three final washes In PBS, the cells were analysed on an Ortho Cytoron (Ortho Diagnostic Systems,

Raritan, NJ, USA) absolute analyser quipped with an argon-ion laser producing 15 mW at 488 nm and a Dell computer running Ortho immunocount software.

10.2.5 Orthotopic (Lung) Xenograft Model for Testing Therapeutic Antibodies

A549 lung adenocarcinoma cells were injected intravenously (2 million cells in 100µl PBS) into nu/nu mice. The mice were sacrificed 60 days later, and 3/4 were found to have multiple tumour colonies in the lung. Based on these findings, a pilot experiment was set up to test the therapeutic effects of mab ICR62. Sixteen nu/nu mice were injected i.v. with 3 million A549 cells. Six were treated with 200µg ICR62 commencing on day 0 and continuing for a total of 11 doses as previously described. Six mice were treated with control mab, and four were untreated. On day 21, two mice from each treatment group were sacrificed and their lungs subjected to histological examination. The remainder were killed on day 60. Tumour growth was assessed semi-quantitatively based on gross and histological examination of lungs. A scoring system was used to describe the extent of tumour growth, since colonies were frequently coalescent and could not always be accurately quantified. In addition, it became clear that only a minority of tumours were growing on the lung surface, so the common practice of counting visible colonies would significantly underestimate tumour growth. The four untreated mice were included in the control group for analytical purposes, but prior to fixation, a total of five tumours from three of the mice were excised under sterile conditions, subjected to enzyme digestion, and the resulting cell suspensions re-established in tissue culture. The cells were analysed by FACS to determine whether their EGFR expression had been modulated by growth in the orthotopic (lung) site. For comparative purposes, A549 cells were also grown s.c, in the spleen, peritoneal cavity and liver of nu/nu mice, and cultured cell lines set up and analysed as before. A thoracic lymph node metastasis found in one of the mice injected with A549 i.p. was also included.

10.2.6 Proliferative Potential of Tumours Explanted Following Treatment with Mabs

Tumours which had responded to therapy were passaged s.c. as fragments via a trocar needle into the flanks of athymic mice to determine their proliferative potential in fresh hosts. Groups of two to eight HN5 or A431 tumours from four separate experiments which had remained static or shown significantly reduced GRs were selected for transplantation. Tumours were measured as before, and the experiments terminated when tumours reached 0.8 cm diameter, or after 60–65 days observation in the absence of progressive growth.

10.3 Results

10.3.1 Response of HN5 Xenografts to Treatment with Anti-EGFR Mabs Commencing on Day 0

Based on in vitro assays, we had established that mabs recognising epitopes C and D were the most effective at inhibiting tumour cell proliferation; whereas a mab recognising epitope A (ICR9) appeared instead to promote ligand binding and growth of EGFR over-expressing carcinoma cells. Figure 1 shows the growth of HN5 carcinomas in mice treated from day 0 with mabs recognising epitopes C and/or D. In mice treated with 200µg doses of ICR62, no tumours were palpable at 7/10 sites by day 7, so treatment was discontinued (total dose administered 1.2 mg). The remaining tumours also rapidly regressed, and no recurrences were observed during an observation period of 90 days. Similarly, complete regressions were obtained with mabs ICR16 (total dose 3 mg) and ICR64 (total dose 2.2 mg). Mabs ICR61 and ICR65 were slightly less effective, in that complete tumour eradication was not achieved. The former resulted in partial regressions, but small nodules remained until the experiment was terminated on day 75, at which point about one third of the tumours were showing some evidence of regrowth. Nine out of ten of the tumours treated with ICR65 remained as small (<2 mm diameter) nodules, and one had grown to 7 mm when the experiment was terminated on day 55. Control mabs had no inhibitory

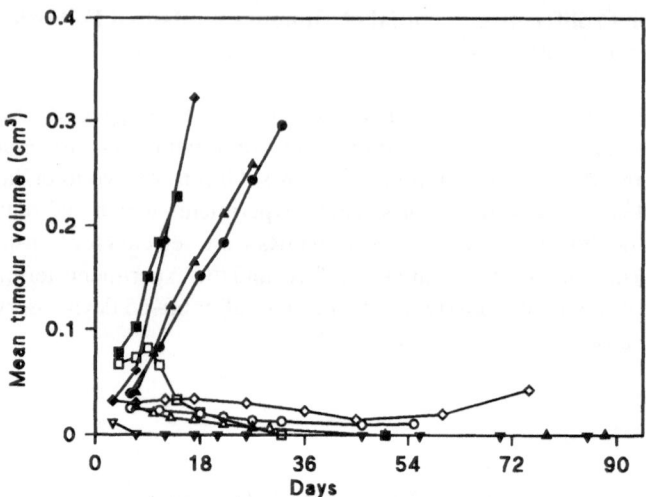

Fig. 1. Inhibitory effects of rat anti- epidermal growth factor receptor mono-
clonal antibodies (mabs) on the growth of HN5 tumor xenografts. Athymic
mice were injected s.c.with 5 million HN5 cells and treated as described in
Sect. 10.2 with 200µg doses of mabs i.p., commencing on the day of tumor
cell inoculation (day 0). Controls: nonspecific IgG1 mab, *solid squares*;
IgG2b, *solid diamond*; IgG2a, *solid triangle*; saline, *solid circle*. Therapy:)
ICR64, *open square*; ICR65, *open circle*; ICR16, *open upright triangle*;
ICR61, *open diamond*; ICR62, *open upside down triangle*

effects on growth compared with saline alone, and the growth curves
reflect the variations obtained between different experiments.

Figure 2 shows a summary of results obtained with these antibodies
where the data are expressed as percentage of control tumour growth. It
serves to indicate the therapeutic efficacy of mabs ICR16, 62 and 64,
and also illustrates the fact that in contrast, tumours in mice given
11×200µg doses of ICR9 exhibited a faster GR than controls.

Since we had achieved complete eradication of HN5 tumour
xenografts with high doses of mabs such as ICR16 and ICR62, we next
tested whether lower doses would be effective. Figure 3 illustrates the
significant growth inhibitory of these mabs when 11 doses of 10µg
(ICR62) or 50µg (ICR16) were given. In the former case, 37.5% of
tumours failed to grow, 25% progressed and the rate of growth of the

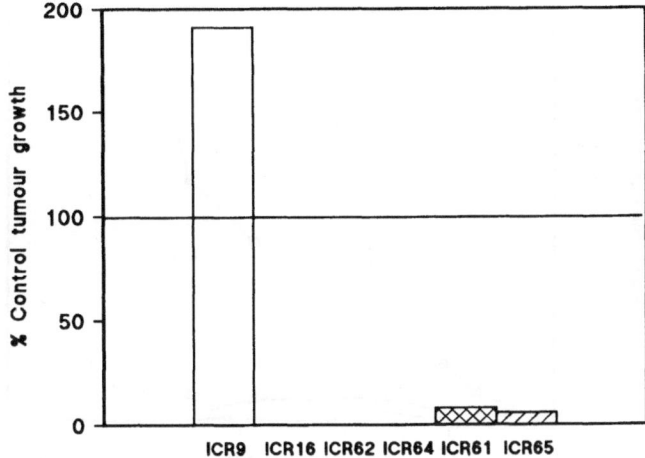

Fig. 2. Summary of the effects of six different anti-epidermal growth factor receptor antibodies on the growth of HN5 tumor xenografts, expressed as per cent control tumour growth. Treatment with 200μg doses commencing on day 0. Schedules as described in the text

remainder was considerably reduced. In the latter case, 25% of tumours regressed completely and the remainder progressed very slowly until the experiment was terminated on day 65. Thus in both cases, treatment with low doses of mab from day 0–18 resulted in long-term control of the majority of HN5 tumours.

10.3.2 Response of Established HN5 Tumours to Therapy with Anti-EGFR Mabs

In the second series of experiments, treatment was delayed until tumours were well established with a mean diameter of 4–6 mm. Figure 4 shows the results obtained with 200μg doses of four different mabs and their appropriate controls. Once again, ICR64 and ICR16 produced excellent therapeutic responses; the former (total 2.2 mg) resulted in 30% complete regressions and 70% static tumours and the latter (total 2.8 mg) 25% complete regressions and 75% static tumours. No tumours

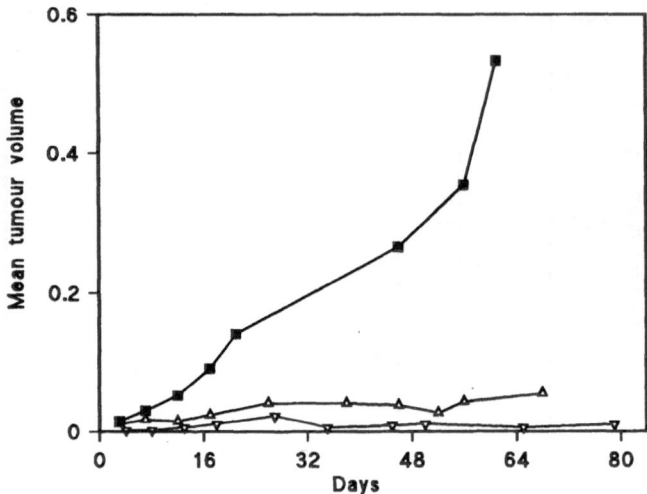

Fig. 3. Effects of low dose treatment with rat anti-epidermal growth factor receptor monoclonal antibodies on the growth of HN5 tumor xenografts.
Athymic mice were injected s.c.with 5 million HN5 cells and treated with
monoclonal antibodies (mabs) from day 0): 10µg doses of ICR62, *open upright triangles*; 50µg doses of ICR16, *open upside down triangles*; 50µg doses
of control mab, *solid squares*. Schedule as described in the text

exhibited progressive growth during observation periods of
75–100 days (Dean et al. 1994).

10.3.2.1 Effects of Varied Treatment Schedules with Mab ICR62 on Growth of Established HN5 Xenografts

We chose mab ICR62 for more detailed studies of differing treatment
schedules, since it had consistently produced excellent results and the
highest percentage of complete regressions even when treating established tumours (Modjtahedi et al. 1993d). We investigated the responses
to limited numbers of higher doses and also lower total doses on the
growth of established tumours. Figure 5 compares the effects of our
original "standard" regime, 11 doses of 200µg given over days 6–24
(group A) with the same total dose (2.2 mg) given as 5×400µg +
1×200µg over days 6–10 (group B). In both cases, tumour regressions

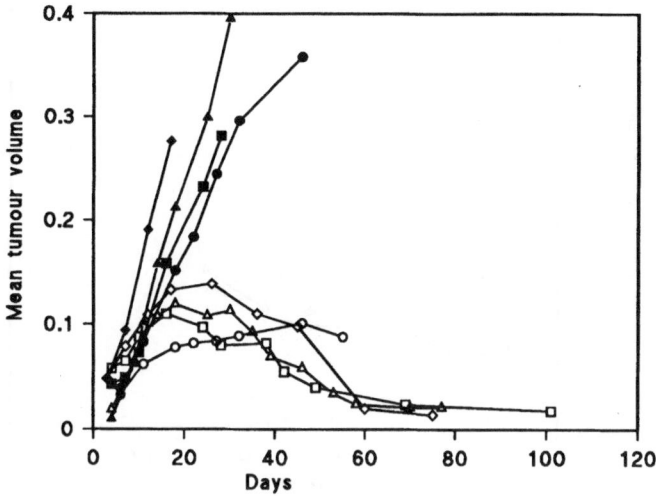

Fig. 4. Inhibitory effects of rat anti-epidermal growth factor receptor mono-clonal antibodies on the growth of established HN5 tumor xenografts. Athymic mice were injected s.c. with 5 million HN5 cells, and treatment was commenced when tumours were 4–5 mm mean diameter (day 5–7). Key as Fig. 1, except that ICR62 is not included

were evident by day 9 and continued until termination of the experiment on day 76 when 40% and 50% (respectively) of sites were tumour free. Control tumours achieved a mean weight of 339 mg by day 24; those in the treated groups were 5.2 (group A) and 2.3 (group B) on day 76. We then compared a single dose of 500μg of ICR62 administered on day 10 (group C) with 5×100μg doses administered between days 10 and 14(group D). The experiment was terminated on day 54 when tumours had achieved mean volumes of 0.14 cm^3(group C) and 0.15 cm^3 (group D) in comparison with controls (not shown) which were a similar size on day 17. GRs were calculated to be 7.01 mg/day in controls compared with 1.91 and 2.7 mg/day for treatment groups C and D, again demonstrating a substantial inhibitory effect of doses of ICR62 approximately one quarter of those employed initially and (in one case) after only a single treatment.

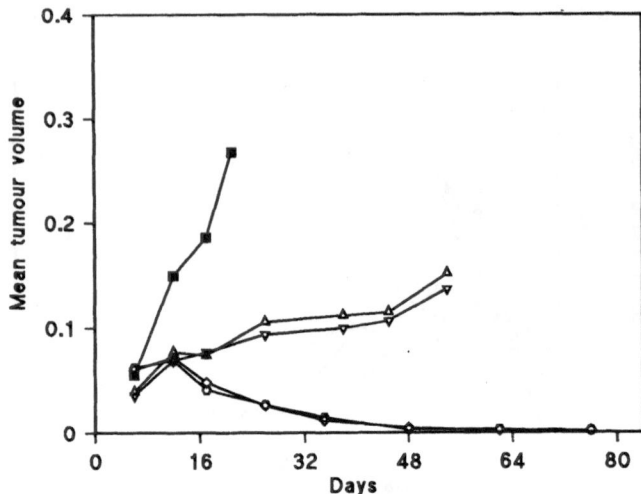

Fig. 5. Effects of varied schedules of treatment with rat monoclonal antibody (mab) ICR62 on the growth of established HN5 xenografts. Tumours were grown s.c. as previously described, and treatment commenced when the tumours were 4–5 mm mean diameter. Key: 11 doses of 200μg, day 6–24, *open diamonds* (group A); five doses of 400μg + one dose of 200μg, day 6–12, *open hexagons* (group B); one dose of 500μg day 10, *open upright triangles* (group C); five doses of 100μg, day 10–14, *open upside down triangles* (group D);.) 11×200μg doses of control mab, *solid squares*

10.3.2.2 Effects of Combinations of Mabs on Growth
of HN5 Xenografts

Since we had available mabs capable of inhibiting tumour growth which recognised two non-cross-reactive epitopes we wished to determine whether therapy with combinations offered advantages compared with single mab therapy. We therefore tested mab ICR62 (epitope C) in combination with ICR61 or ICR64 (epitope D) on established HN5 xenografts. We found that 11 doses of 100μg of each mab (combined total 2.2 mg) was no more effective than equivalent doses of monotherapy (Modjtahedi et al. 1993e). A similar lack of synergy was observed in vitro with all combinations of mabs tested. The relative in vivo efficacy (expressed as per cent control tumour growth) of all the mabs

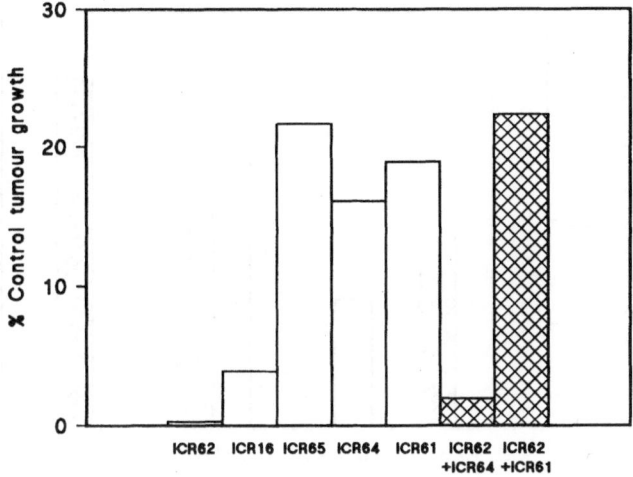

Fig. 6. Summary of the effects of five different anti-epidermal growth factor receptor antibodies plus two combination therapies on the growth of established HN5 tumor xenografts. Treatment schedules as described in the text

tested against established HN5 tumours is illustrated in Fig. 6, where once again ICR62 gave the best results.

10.3.2.3 Effects of Anti-EGFR Mabs
on Different Human Tumour Xenografts

HN5 (derived from a squamous cell carcinoma of the head and neck) has particularly high levels of EGFR, and it was important to examine the therapeutic effects of our mabs on tumours of other tissue types and also those with more modest levels of over-expression of EGFR (Table 2).

Figure 7 summarises the effects of our "standard" therapy regime (11×200µg doses) of ICR62 and ICR16 on four different human tumour xenografts (except in the case of MDA MB 468 where doses of only 20µg were used). In each case, where tested, ICR16 was less effective than ICR62. Complete regressions of the breast carcinoma MDA MB 468 were obtained with ICR62, and growth inhibitions of between 16% (A172) and 63% (A431). In the latter case 40% of tumours regressed completely (Modjtahedi et al. 1993d). We also found that ICR62 (11×200µg) could induce substantial growth inhibition of established

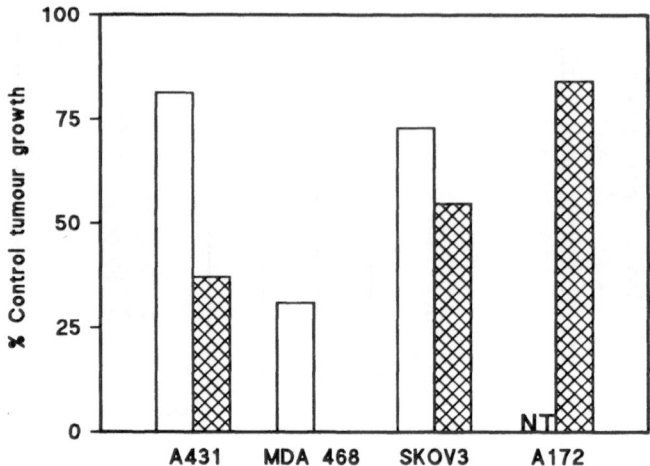

Fig. 7. Summary of the effects of anti-epidermal growth factor receptor antibodies ICR16 and ICR62 on the growth of four different human tumor xenografts. Treatment commenced on day 0, schedules as described in the text. ICR16, *open bars*; ICR62, *hatched bars*

breast carcinoma xenografts (12.5% complete regressions and 75% stable disease: data not shown).

10.3.2.4 Histological Examination
of Tumours Undergoing Regression

We routinely fixed and stained any residual tumour nodules at the termination of therapy with anti-EGFR mabs, and in most cases little viable tumour tissue remained. Figure 8 illustrates the histological appearance of HN5 xenografts treated with control mab (group A) or ICR9 (group B)(which caused growth enhancement) from day 0–18. The cells appear viable, there is little if any necrosis, and particularly in the latter, mitotic figures are visible. The appearance of tumours following treatment with single mabs or combinations is represented in Fig. 8c,d. Of note is the appearance of keratinised areas suggestive of squamous cell differentiation and the lack of viable tumour cells. This characteristic appearance of regressing HN5 tumours was found with all growth inhibitory mabs or mab combinations tested and was not unique to a

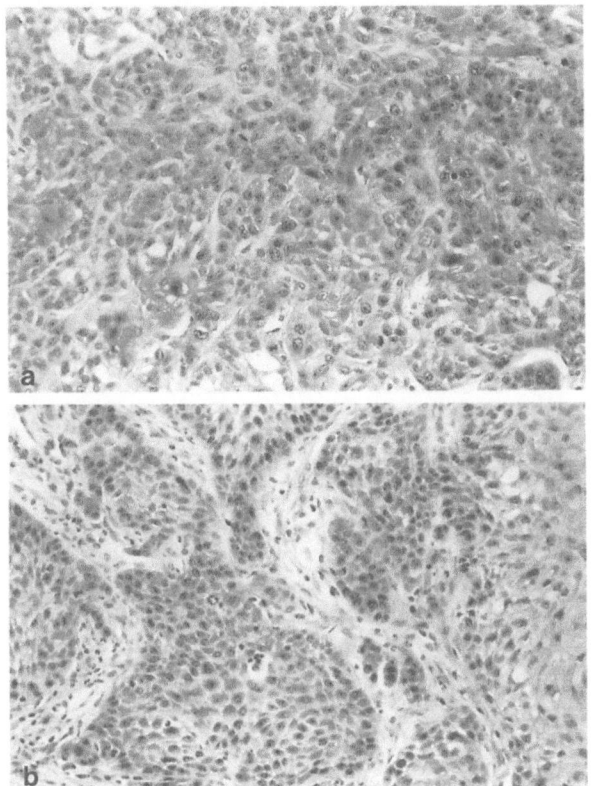

Fig. 8a–d. Haematoxylin and eosin stained fixed tissue sections of HN5 tumor xenografts ×200. Mice treated with 200μg doses of control monoclonal antibody, tumour taken day 27 (**a**); ICR9, day 21 (**b**); ICR61, day 75 (**c**); ICR62+ICR64, day 79. Treatments in **a** and **b** from day 0–18; treatments **c** and **d** from day 7–24 (**d**). **c,d** see p. 200

particular mab. These observations suggested that terminal differentiation may be an important consequence of the therapeutic effects of these anti-EGFR mabs.

MDA MB 468 tumours treated with therapeutic mabs appeared largely necrotic, with pyknotic nuclei and apoptotic bodies present in some areas (Modjtahedi et al. 1994). There was no evidence of glandular differentiation, suggesting that the response to growth inhibitory mabs

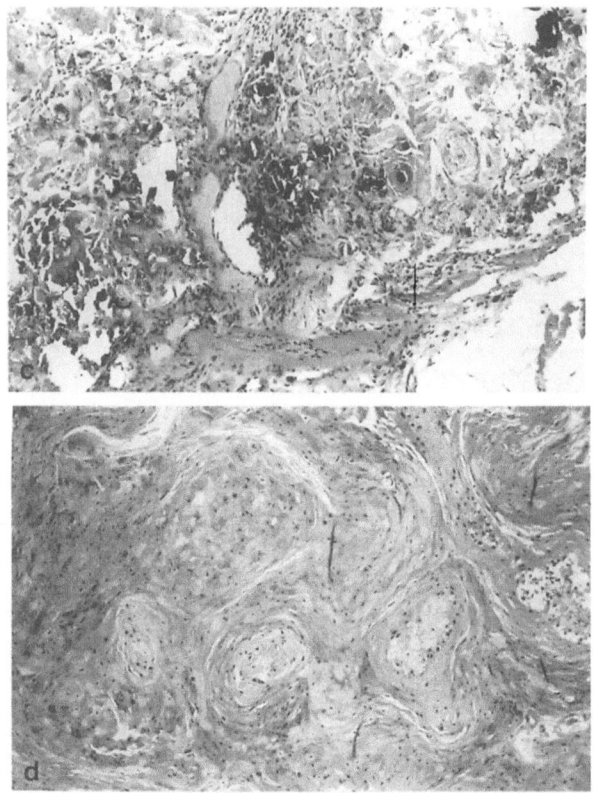

Fig. 8c,d. Legend see p. 199

of EGFR over-expressing tumours derived from squamous and secretory epithelia may be qualitatively different.

We next investigated earlier events in HN5 tumour regression, since
the late events seemed to be common to all therapeutic mabs tested and
did not explain the discrepancy between, for example ICR16 and
ICR62, where the former is more effective in tumour cell growth inhibition in vitro, but is less effective than the latter in vivo (Modjtahedi et al.
1993b–d). Figure 9 illustrates frozen sections of HN5 tumours sampled
7 days after cell inoculation following five doses of ICR16 (group A) or
ICR62 (group B). The sections have been stained with an immunoper-

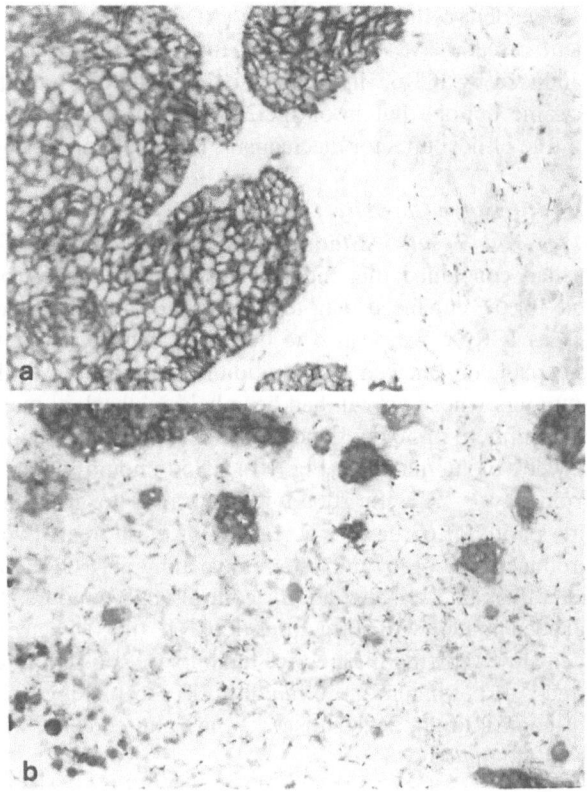

Fig. 9a,b. Sections of HN5 tumor xenografts (×200) 7 days after inoculation of 5 million cells s.c. in athymic mice treated with 5´200μg of ICR16 (**a**) and treated with 5×200μg ICR62 (**b**) on days 0–4. Tumours were cryosectioned and stained directly with immunoperoxidase-conjugated F(abÆ)2 rabbit anti-rat Ig antibody to detect bound primary antibodies

oxidase-conjugated rabbit anti-rat IG reagent to visualise the presence of the therapeutic mabs. In both cases there is extensive localisation of the mabs on the tumour cell membranes, but in the latter case the tumour foci are smaller and more fragmentary and surrounded by extensive host cell infiltrates. ICR62 is a rat IgG2b mab, and it is known that this isotype is capable of recruiting Fc-receptor-bearing host cells to mediate antibody-dependent cellular cytotoxicity (ADCC) and in activating the complement cascade. We speculate that the more rapid regression of tumours induced by ICR62 in comparison with ICR16 (which recognises the same epitope but is of IgG2a isotype) may be due to the additional role of host effector mechanisms (Modjtahedi et al. 1994).

10.3.2.5 Proliferative Capacity
of Explanted Mab-Treated "Static" Tumours

Since we had concluded that induced host responses may be partly responsible for the enhanced long-term control of tumours treated with mabs such as ICR62, we wished to determine whether such tumours would be capable of renewed proliferation in naive hosts. We therefore selected tumours whose growth had been held in check in mab-treated hosts for a minimum of 50 days and transplanted them as fragments s.c. in fresh 5-week-old nu/nu mice (Fig. 10). HN5 tumours which had been treated from day 6–24 with 200µg ICR62 failed to grow during an observation period of 63 days; whereas 3/4 of those treated with 10µg ICR62 produced slow-growing progressive tumours (GR=3.73 compared with values of 8–14 mg/day for control HN5 tumours. Tumours which had been treated with 50µg doses of ICR16 (n=8) when explanted also yielded slow-growing progressive tumours (GR=3.43). In contrast, transplanted A431 tumours grew rapidly (GR=26 mg/day), similar to the rate of control tumours established from cultured cells, which was generally 14–20 mg/day.

10.3.2.6 Response of Orthotopic Lung Carcinoma Xenografts
to Treatment with Mab ICR62

Mice which had been injected i.v. with A549 lung carcinoma cells and treated with ICR62 or control mab (200µg×11 from day 0–18) were killed on day 21 or 60 following inoculation. At the early time point, 2/2 control mice already showed evidence of multiple microscopic tumour colonies, whereas no tumour was detectable in ICR62 treated mice. On day 60, 7/8 control mice had extensive lung tumour development (4/8 with more than 50 gross colonies), and the remaining mouse had multiple microscopic colonies and three gross colonies. In contrast, one ICR62-treated mouse had no evidence of malignant disease, two had microscopic disease only, and the fourth had approximately 20–25 gross colonies. This preliminary small scale study suggests that the orthotopic

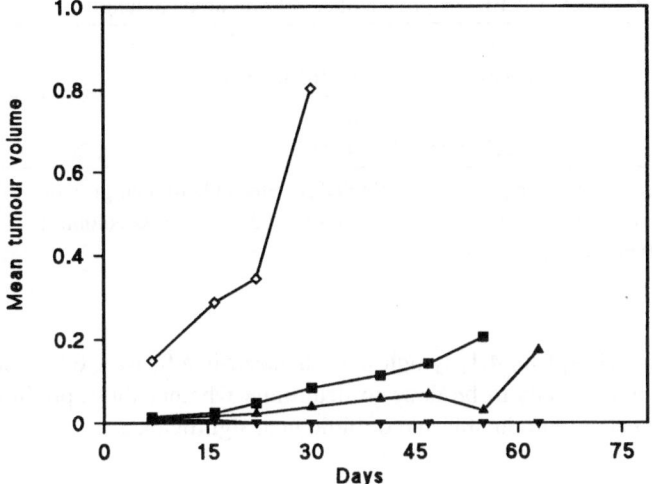

Fig. 10. Transplantation and fate of tumours explanted following treatment with rat anti-epidermal growth factor receptor monoclonal antibodies. Tumours which had responded to therapy were passaged s.c. as fragments into the flanks of further athymic mice to determine their proliferative potential in the absence of further treatment.) HN5 tumours treated with 11 doses of 200μg ICR62 taken at day 76 following cell inoculation (*n=2*), *solid upside down triangles*; HN5 tumours treated with 10μg ICR62 taken at day 57 (*n=4*), *solid upright triangles*; HN5 tumours treated with 11 doses of 50μg ICR16 taken at day 68 (*n=8*), *solid squares*; A431 tumour treated with 200μg ICR62 taken at day 51 (*n=4*), *open diamonds*

site may be an appropriate and sensitive test system in which to analyse the therapeutic effects of mabs, particularly where EGFR over-expression is modest, as in the case of A549. Such tumours (see also results with A172 and SKOV 3, Table 2 and Fig. 7) rarely respond well when grown at subcutaneous sites.

When we checked the EGFR expression levels in A549 cells by FACS analysis following their growth in vivo, we were interested to find that the mean fluorescence intensity had increased in the explanted lung tumours (from 2.5 in the controls to between 7.6 and 16.3 in five separate cell lines). A549 sublines derived from growth at other sites showed a less marked increase in fluorescence intensity (s.c. 4.9; i.p

Table 3. Effect of ICR62 on growth of A549 carcinoma in lung

Day	Tumour growth Control	ICR62 treated
21	1;1	0;0
60	1;2;2;2;3;3;3;3	0;1;1;2

Scoring grade:0, No gross or histologically detectable tumour growth;
1, Microscopic colonies or < 5 gross colonies; 2, 5–50 gross colonies;
3, > 50 gross colonies

ascites 3.1; spleen 4.1; lymph node metastasis 4.9; liver 6.5). Clearly
more work needs to be done to determine whether these preliminary
findings are reproducible and of biological significance.

10.4 Discussion

Our approach of using a variety of tumour systems to both generate and
test the activity of rat mabs to human EGFR has yielded some interesting observations. Firstly, as predicted, we were able to generate a large
number of mabs with diverse properties which have enabled us to
dissect important principles determining biological response and to
select the best mab overall for future development. Without exception,
mabs which bound to epitopes C and D were the most effective at
inhibiting ligand binding and mitogenic signal transduction in vitro,
whilst mabs recognising epitope A seemed rather to potentiate the
effects of ligand–receptor interactions. However, those antibodies which
were the most potent in vitro (based on IC_{50} values) were not necessarily those which had the greatest therapeutic effects in vivo. In general,
mabs of IgG2b isotype were more effective than those of the same
epitope preference but of IgG2a isotype (e.g. ICR62:ICR16). These data
are consistent with earlier studies using mouse IgG2a mabs (which like
rat IgG2b can recruit Fc-receptor-bearing host cells and activate complement) where host-mediated effects contributed significantly to the
therapeutic effects obtained (Masui et al. 1986; Rodeck et al. 1987).

Examination of histological sections of tumours undergoing regression confirmed the presence of significant host cell infiltration at early

stages following treatment with ICR62. In residual HN5 lesions which persisted following treatment of established tumours with therapeutic mabs, the presence of keratinised areas suggested that the cells may have been induced to undergo terminal differentiation. This was confirmed in in vitro studies in which we showed that expression of the specific keratinocyte differentiation markers cytokeratin 10 and involucrin was inducible in HN5 cells by mabs which inhibited their growth (Modjtahedi et al. 1994; Modjatahedi and Dean 1995a). Further work also showed that monovalent Fab fragments of ICR62 at 25μg/ml could inhibit the growth and direct the terminal differentiation of HN5 as effectively as intact mab (Modjtahedi et al. 1995). Thus, although we have not yet tested the activity of mab fragments in vivo, these data encourage the view that such constructs should be active, and their more rapid extravasation may be of advantage in gaining access to disseminated disease. Studies by Nair et al. (1994) have shown that interferon β can also induce terminal differentiation in vitro of NCI-H596 adenosquamous lung carcinoma cells, and the sequence of events suggested a causal relationship between differentiation induction and subsequent growth suppression. It will be of interest to determine whether the underlying molecular mechanisms are common to both agents.

The response of different tumours to EGFR blockade appears to be the result of a complex interplay between levels of this receptor, the degree of dependence on EGFR signalling versus other ligand-receptor pathways, and the ability of the cell to produce its own (autocrine) ligands. Comparison of the ability of the mabs to control the growth of different human tumour xenografts showed that, as expected, those with higher levels of EGFR over-expression (such as HN5 and MDA MB 468) were more responsive than those with lower levels (e.g. A172 and A549). Cells like A431 which shed a truncated receptor and/or secrete large amounts of transforming growth factor-α (TGFα) were less responsive than might be expected from their EGFR density, and also were able to grow out after cessation of mab therapy if complete control was not achieved (e.g. with ICR16), whereas HN5 tumours in most cases remained static, and did not resume progressive growth even when transplanted to fresh hosts (Fig. 10).

Clearly, human tumours are likely to present a wide spectrum of EGFR expression and dependency, and, in addition to producing the best library of mabs for therapy, we should consider combination ap-

Table 4. Phase 1 localisation trial of ICR62 in patients with squamous cell carcinoma

Patients (*n*)	Mab dose (mg)	Toxicity (WHO grade)	HARA
3	2.5	0–II	–
3	10	I	–
3	20	I–II	1/3 anti-id
3	40	I	1/3 anti-i
8	100	I–II	2/8

proaches. Interestingly, therapy with two mabs given together gave no advantages compared with the best mab (ICR62) given alone (Fig. 6). However, availability of more than one effective mab may prove of benefit for sequential therapy if patients mount anti-idiotypic responses to primary mab therapy. Also, since when different tumours were used as immunogens, mabs recognising different epitopes were obtained (Table 1), it is possible that expression of the four epitopes we have defined (and possibly others as yet undiscovered) may vary between tumours of different histogenic origin. The possibility that EGFR expression may vary in response to microenvironmental influences must also be taken into consideration. The importance of orthotopic human tumour xenograft models is gradually becoming apparent (Eccles et al. 1994). The ability of human colon carinoma cells to grow in the liver of nu/nu mice was recently shown to correlate with five- to tenfold enhanced EGFR expression (Radinsky 1995), and site-dependent variations in expression of cellular antigens, multidrug resistance markers and other biological traits have been frequently reported. In the present study, A549 lung adenocarcinoma cells grown orthotopically provided a fairly sensitive assay system to detect therapeutic effects of anti-EGFR mabs and on explant were found to have receptor levels up-regulated by 3–6.5-fold. Tumours grown at other sites did not show the same overall level of EGFR enhancement, but interestingly those grown in the liver showed the greatest increase (2.6-fold).

A few previous studies have attempted to test the therapeutic effects of anti-EGFR mabs against tumours grown at orthotopic or metastatic sites. For example, Naramura et al. (1993) showed that m225 anti-EGFR mab was capable of inhibiting metastasis of M24met melanoma in SCID mice solely by activating immune effector cells, and Aboud-Pirak et al. (1988) showed that mab 108.4 reduced the number of lung colonies produced by KB oral epidermoid carcinoma to 15% of control values. Clearly, the further development of these and similar models – including perhaps the generation of mice transgenic for human EGFR to assess effects on normal tissues which express this receptor – will provide more sophisticated systems for the preclinical evaluation of mabs and their constructs.

The mabs described in this paper have demonstrated growth inhibitory effects against a variety of human tumour xenografts which compare favourably with those previously reported. Early results from a clinical trial with mab ICR62 have proved encouraging, and we are actively developing this molecule for clinical use. The recognition of deletion-mutant forms of EGFR, firstly in brain malignancies and more recently in other tumour types (Wikstrand et al. 1995), is also an interesting finding which may enable the development of truly "tumour-specific" mabs for some subsets of patients.

References

Aboud-Pirak E, Hurwitz E, Pirak ME, Bellot F, Schlessinger J, Sela M (1988) Efficacy of antibodies to epidermal growth factor against KB carcinoma in vitro and in nude mice. J Natl Cancer Inst 80:1605–1611

Baselga J, Mendelsohn J (1994) The epidermal growth factor receptor as a target for therapy in breast carcinoma. Breast Cancer Res Treat 29:127–138

Dean C, Modjtahedi H, Eccles S, Box G, Styles J (1994) Immunotherapy with antibodies to the EGF receptor. Int J Cancer [Suppl] 8:103–107

Eccles S, Box G, Court W, Sandle J, Dean CJ (1994) Preclinical models for the evaluation of targeted therapies of metastatic disease. Cell Biophys 24/25:279–291

Eccles S, Modjtahedi H, Box G, Court W, Sandle J, Dean C (1995) Significance of the c-erbB family of receptor tyrosine kinases in metastatic cancer and their potential as targets for immunotherapy. Invasion Metastasis 14:337–348

Harris AL, Nicholson S, Sainsbury R, Wright C, Farndon J (1992) Epidermal growth factor receptor and other oncogenes as prognostic markers. J Natl Cancer Inst Monogr 11:181–188

Khaziae K, Schirrmacher V, Lichtner RB (1993) EGF receptor in neoplasia and metastasis. Cancer Metastasis Rev 12:255–274

Masui H, Moroyama T, Mendelsohn J (1986) Mechanism of antitumour activity in mice for anti-epidermal growth factor antibodies with different isotypes. Cancer Res 46:5592–5598

Modjtahedi H, Dean C (1994) The receptor for EGF and its ligands: expression, prognostic value and target for therapy in cancer (review). Int J Oncol 4:227–296

Modjtahedi H, Dean C (1995a) Antibody-induced inhibition of EGFR overexpressing tumours occurs in the absence of receptor down-regulation. Int J Oncol 7:783–788

Modjtahedi H, Dean C (1995b) The binding of HB-EGF to tumour cells is blocked by mabs which act as EGF and TGFα antagonists. Biochem Biophys Res Commun 207:389–397

Modjtahedi H, Styles J, Dean CJ (1993a) The growth response of human tumour cell lines expressing the EGF receptor to treatment with EGF and/or Mabs that block ligand binding. Int J Oncol 3:237–243

Modjtahedi H, Styles J, Box G, Eccles S, Gusterson B, Dean C (1993b) Antitumour activity of rat Mabs to the human receptor for EGF. In: Epenetos AA, Lemoine NR (eds) Mutant oncogenes: targets for therapy? Chapman and Hall, London, p 35

Modjtahedi H, Styles JM, Dean CJ (1993c) The human EGF receptor as a target for cancer therapy: six new rat mAbs against the receptor on breast carcinoma MDA-MB 468. Br J Cancer 67:247–253

Modjtahedi H, Eccles S, Box G, Styles J, Dean C (1993d) Immunotherapy of human tumour xenografts overexpressing the EGF receptor with rat antibodies that block growth factor-receptor interaction. Br J Cancer 67:254–261

Modjtahedi H, Eccles SA, Box G, Styles J, Dean CJ (1993e) Antitumor activity of combinations of antibodies directed against different epitopes on the extacellular domain of the human EGF receptor. Cell Biophys 22:129–146

Modjtahedi H, Eccles S, Sandle J, Box G, Titley J Dean C (1994) Differentiation or immune destruction: two pathways for therapy of squamous cell carcinomas with antibodies to the epidermal growth factor receptor. Cancer Res 54:1695–1701

Modjtahedi H, Jackson E, Dean C (1995) Monovalent antibodies to the epidermal growth factor (EGF) receptor: effects on proliferation and differentiation of tumors overexpressing the EGF receptor. Tumor Target 1:99–106

Modjtahedi H, Hickish T, Nicolson M, Moore J, Styles J, Eccles S, Jackson E, Salter J, Sloane J, Spencer L, Priest K, Smith I, Dean C, Gore M (1996) Phase 1 trial and tumour localisation of the anti-EGFR monoclonal antibody ICR62 in head and neck or lung cancer. Br J Cancer 73:228–235

Nair S, Mayotte J, Lockshin A, Levitt M (1994) Induction of squamous differentiation by interferonβ in a human non-small cell lung cancer cell line. J Natl Cancer Inst 86:378–383

Naramura M, Gillies SD, Mendelsohn J, Reisfeld RA, Mueller B (1993) Therapeutic potential of chimeric and murine anti-(epidermal growth factor receptor) antibodies in a metastasis model for human melanoma. Cancer Immunol Immunother 37:343–349

Radinsky R (1995) Molecular mechanisms for organ-specific colon carcinoma metastasis. Eur J Cancer 31A:1091–1095

Rodeck U, Herlyn, M, Herlyn D, Molthoff C, Atkinson B, Varello M, Steplewski Z, Koprowski H (1987) Tumor growth modulation by a monoclonal antibody to the epidermal growth factor receptor: immunologically mediated and effector cell-independent effects. Cancer Res 47:3692–3696

Sato JD, Le AD, Kawamoto T (1987) Derivation and assay of biological effects of monoclonal antibodies to epidermal growth factor receptors. Methods Enzymol 146:63–81

Wikstrand C, Hale LP, Batra SK et al (1995) Monoclonal antibodies against EGFRvIII are tumor specific and react with breast and lung carcinomas and malignant gliomas. Cancer Res 55:3140–3148

11 Recombinant Fusion Toxins Targeted to Members of the ErbB Family of Receptor Tyrosine Kinases

W. Wels, M. Schmidt, M. Jeschke, B. Groner, R.R. Beerli,
N.E. Hynes, and M. Hoffmann

11.1 Introduction

More than a decade ago, cytotoxic agents termed immunotoxins were designed by coupling bacterial or plant toxins to monoclonal antibodies specific for molecules on the surface of tumor cells. Advances in various fields of investigation have led to refined approaches and a new generation of recombinant toxin constructs are currently being tested in cancer therapy. The new strategies still employ the two original principles: (1) they rely on the enhanced expression of cell surface molecules in tumor cells when compared to normal cells, and (2) they utilize bifunctional molecules combining a tumor cell recognition domain and a toxic domain.

The elucidation of the molecular structure and the functional domains of bacterial toxins such as diphtheria toxin from *Corynebacterium diphtheriae* and exotoxin A from *Pseudomonas aeruginosa* has allowed these molecules to be miniaturized through recombinant DNA techniques and to produce them as single polypeptides in large quantities and of consistent quality in bacteria. Proteins with novel target cell specificity are produced by replacing the original cell-binding domain of such toxins with peptide hormones, growth factors, or cytokines (reviewed in Pastan and FitzGerald 1991). With the advent of recombinant antibody technology single-chain derivatives of monoclonal antibodies (scFv, molecular fusions of the variable domains of the heavy and light chains) have been used as alternative recognition domains. These single-chain immunotoxins are much smaller than the original chemical conjugates of monoclonal antibodies and toxins and have superior properties regarding their penetration of large tumors.

An important prerequisite for the therapeutic application of immunotoxins is the identification of suitable antigens on the surface of tumor cells. The exclusive or enhanced expression of the target molecule on tumor cells has to be demonstrated. The erbB/EGF receptor-related gene family encodes growth factor receptors with intrinsic tyrosine kinase activity. Four members of this family have been identified: ErbB/EGF receptor, ErbB-2/HER2/Neu, ErbB-3 and ErbB-4 (reviewed in Peles and Yarden 1993). Members of this family have been implicated in the development of a variety of human malignancies. Overexpression of EGF receptor and ErbB-2 has been observed in a high percentage of primary human adenocarcinomas and correlates with an unfavorable prognosis for the patient (reviewed in Gullick 1991; Hynes and Stern 1994). Increased expression of ErbB-3 and ErbB-4 has also been found in a subset of human mammary tumors and in several established tumor cell lines, respectively (Lemoine et al. 1992; Plowman et al. 1993). Due to their preferential expression in tumor cells, their accessibility from the extracellular space, and their involvement in the transformation process the ErbB/EGF receptor-related tyrosine kinases may be regarded as appropriate targets for cytotoxic molecules which preferentially attack tumor cells.

11.2 Derivation of ErbB-2
and EGF Receptor-Specific Single-Chain Antibodies

Monoclonal antibodies (MAb) directed against the extracellular domain of the ErbB-2 protein have been described by different groups. Some of these antibodies inhibit the in vitro or in vivo growth of tumor cells when tested alone (Hudziak et al. 1989; Stancovski et al. 1991; Harwerth et al. 1992) or in combination (Kasprzyk et al. 1992; Harwerth et al. 1993). Recent advances in the field of molecular immunology have made it possible to utilize antibody-derived binding domains for the target cell-specific delivery of therapeutic effector functions (Winter and Milstein 1991). From a panel of MAbs which specifically recognize the ErbB-2 protein (Harwerth et al. 1992) we have derived recombinant scFv molecules. They consist of the variable domains of the antibody heavy and light chains connected via a flexible linker sequence (Wels et al. 1992a). RNA isolated from hybridoma cells was used to prime first strand cDNA synthesis of the light chain and heavy chain transcripts. Subsequently, the cDNAs were amplified by polymerase chain reaction (PCR) using oligonucleotides designed to match consensus sequences deduced from a collection of known immunoglobulin cDNA sequences at the 5' and 3' ends of the rearranged light (VL) and heavy (VH) chain variable regions. The amplified cDNA sequences were joined into one open reading frame using a linker coding for the 15 amino acids (Gly, Gly, Gly, Gly, Ser)$_3$ (Wels et al. 1992a). This amino acid linker allows the correct folding of the antigen-binding domain in the recombinant molecule.

The resulting scFv-encoding gene fragments were introduced into a vector suitable for the expression of recombinant proteins in *Escherichia coli*. Recombinant antibodies purified from bacterial extracts are able to bind to ErbB-2 with high affinity. This was demonstrated by immunoprecipitation of scFv–ErbB-2 complexes from a mixture of scFv molecules derived from MAbs FRP5 and FWP51 with tumor cell lysates containing the ErbB-2 protein (Wels et al. 1992a). In order to test the capacity of the scFv domain to direct an effector function specifically to ErbB-2-expressing tumor cells, the FRP5 derived antibody gene fragment was fused to the bacterial alkaline phosphatase gene phoA. The resulting phosphatase fusion protein carrying the scFv domain at the N-terminus is enzymatically active and binds specifically to ErbB-2-expressing cells, indicating that this molecule is bifunctional (Wels et al. 1992c). Due to its superior activity, the scFv(FRP5) molecule was chosen as a binding domain in several approaches aimed at the targeted interference with tumor cell growth via the ErbB-2 protein (Wels et al. 1992b; Moritz et al. 1994; Beerli et al. 1994a).

Similarly a scFv antibody molecule with specificity for the EGF receptor was derived by recombinant DNA techniques from the hybridoma cell line producing MAb 225 (Kawamoto et al. 1983). The biological characteristics of the MAb 225 have been studied in great detail by John Mendelsohn and colleagues. MAb 225 competes with epidermal growth factor (EGF) for binding to the EGF receptor, thereby blocking ligand-dependent receptor activation (Fan et al. 1993). Treatment with MAb 225 inhibits the growth of EGF receptor-expressing tumor cells in vitro and in vivo (Masui et al. 1984; Ennis et al. 1989). Bacterially expressed scFv(225) protein like the parental MAb specifically binds to the human EGF receptor, thereby blocking its activation by EGF (Wels et al. 1995a). Intracellular expression of a scFv(225) derivative carrying an immunoglobulin signal peptide resulted in the inhibition of the EGF-dependent growth in soft agar of murine fibroblasts transfected with human EGF receptor cDNA, presumably via an autocrine mechanism (Beerli et al. 1994b).

11.3 Construction of Recombinant Antibody and Growth Factor Toxins

Exotoxin A (ETA) from *Pseudomonas aeruginosa* is a potent inhibitor of protein synthesis in mammalian cells. The 66-kDa protein consists of three functional domains: an N-terminal cell-binding domain Ia, an internal translocation domain II, and a C-terminal enzymatic domain III which facilitates the ADP-ribosylation of eukaryotic elongation factor 2. After binding to target cells ETA is internalized. In the acidic environment of the endosome a conformational change occurs, the toxin is proteolytically cleaved within its translocation domain and the C-terminal effector domain translocates to the cytosol (Zdanovsky et al. 1993). Members of the ErbB family of receptor tyrosine kinases present suitable targets for ETA-derived fusion toxins. Molecules binding to the

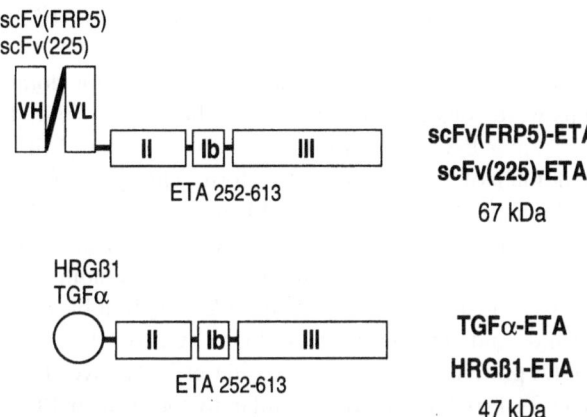

Fig. 1. Schematic structure of recombinant single-chain toxins. The bacterially expressed antibody toxins scFv(FRP5)-ETA and scFv(225)-ETA consist of the scFv domain of the monoclonal antibodies FRP5 specific for ErbB-2, and 225 specific for the EGF receptor containing the heavy (*VH*) and light chain (*VL*) variable domains, fused to amino acids 252 to 613 of *Pseudomonas* exotoxin A (*ETA*). The toxin fragment represents the translocation domain *II*, domain *Ib*, and domain *III* which mediates the ADP ribosylation of the eukaryotic elongation factor 2. The growth factor toxins HRGβ1-ETA and TGF-α-ETA contain the epidermal growth factor (EGF)-like domain of the ErbB-3/ErbB-4 ligand heregulin β1 (amino acids 177 to 246 of the parental molecule) or amino acids 1 to 50 of the EGF receptor ligand transforming growth factor-α (*TGF-α*), respectively. Included in the molecules are the *E. coli* ompA signal peptide, a synthetic 8 amino acids epitope (FLAG epitope) and a cluster of six His residues at the N-terminus, and a cluster of six His residues N-terminal of the ETA domain II facilitating the purification of the proteins via Ni^{2+} and immunoaffinity chromatography (not shown)

extracellular domain of such receptors can be internalized via normal receptor turnover or ligand-induced internalization which allows the activation of the toxin moiety. A truncated ETA gene, encoding amino acids 252 to 613, and lacking the original cell-binding domain Ia was derived by PCR mutagenesis and fused to the 3' end of the scFv(FRP5) and scFv(225) genes in a bacterial expression vector (Wels et al. 1992b, 1995a). Recombinant proteins were expressed in *E. coli* and purified from bacterial extracts via affinity chromatography. The structure of the resulting 67-kDa single chain antibody toxins scFv(FRP5)-ETA and scFv(225)-ETA is shown schematically in Fig. 1.

Likewise, fusion toxins which carry a growth factor domain at the N-terminus were constructed. cDNAs encoding amino acids 1 to 50 of the EGF receptor ligand transforming growth factor-α (TGF-α) or the EGF-like domain of the heregulin β1 isoform (HRGβ1, amino acids 177 to 246) which binds ErbB-3 and ErbB-4 (Tzahar et al. 1994) were derived by reverse transcription of mRNA isolated from, respectively, MDA-MB468 and MDA-MB231 human breast carcinoma cells. These sequences were fused to the truncated ETA gene in a bacterial expression plasmid and recombinant 47-kDa TGF-α-ETA and 48-kDa HRGβ1-ETA proteins were produced as described above (Jeschke et al. 1995). The TGF-α-ETA is very similar to the TGF-α-PE40 protein previously described by others (Siegall et al. 1989).

The ability of the heterologous binding domains of the recombinant toxins to recognize their target receptors was analyzed. ScFv(FRP5)-ETA and scFv(225)-ETA displayed apparent binding affinities of 4.2 and 12 nM, respectively, in enzyme-linked immunosorbent assay (ELISA) experiments using EGF receptor overexpressing MDA-MB468 or ErbB-2 overexpressing SKBR3 breast tumor cells (Wels et al. 1995a). The binding of HRGβ1-ETA was analyzed using MDA-MB453 cells which express high levels of ErbB-2, ErbB-3 and ErbB-4. Upon short-term treatment of the cells with HRGβ1-ETA immunoblots with a phosphotyrosine antibody showed an increase in the phosphotyrosine content of a protein of approximately 185 kDa (Jeschke et al. 1995). A similar increase was observed in cells treated with the heregulin homologue neu differentiation factor (NDF) but was not observed in cells treated with the ErbB-2 specific scFv(FRP5)-ETA molecule. Similarly, treatment of A431 squamous carcinoma cells with the TGF-α-ETA protein led to an increase in the phosphotyrosine content of a 170-kDa protein which was identified as the EGF receptor (Schmidt and Wels, unpublished observation). This indicates that the growth factor toxins retain the ability to recognize the appropriate receptor molecules.

11.4 Functional Characterization of Recombinant Toxins In Vitro

The specificity and cytotoxic activity of the antibody and growth factor toxins was determined in cell viability assays in vitro. Several human tumor cell lines expressing different levels of the four ErbB receptor family members were treated with various concentrations of ETA fusion toxins and the fraction of surviving cells was determined using an enzymatic assay as described (Wels et al. 1992b). The scFv(FRP5)-ETA and scFv(225)-ETA proteins were very potent in the inhibition of tumor cell growth and highly selective for tumor cells overexpressing ErbB-2 or the EGF receptor, respectively, with IC_{50} values ranging from 2 to 200 ng/ml (Wels et al. 1992b, 1995a) (pM order of magnitude, summarized in Table 1). MDA-MB468 cells, which overexpress the EGF receptor but have less than 5000 ErbB-2 molecules, were sensitive to scFv(225)-ETA but were not affected by scFv(FRP5)-ETA even at high

Table 1. Cytotoxic activity of ETA fusion proteins on human tumor cells in vitro

Cell line	MDA-MB468	A431	SKBR3	MDA-MB453	T47D
Relative level of receptor expression					
EGFR	+++++	+++++	+	+/–	+
ErbB-2	+/–	+	++++	++++	++
ErbB-3	n.d.	+	+++	++++	+++
ErbB-4	n.d.	–	–	+++	+++
Toxin	IC_{50} (nM)				
HRGβ1-ETA[a]	n.d.	5.94	0.12	0.08	0.99
TGFα-ETA	0.02	<0.02	1.66	0.53	2.23
scFv(225)-ETA[b]	2.27	0.07	>15	n.d.	>15
scFv(FRP5)-ETA[b,c]	>15	0.52	0.34	<0.01	0.13

The 50% inhibitory concentrations were determined in an enzymatic cell viability assay.

n.d., not done.

[a]Jeschke et al. 1995.

[b]Wels et al. 1995a.

[c]Wels et al. 1992b.

doses. Similarly, SKBR3 cells which overexpress ErbB-2 and have approximately 9×10^4 EGF receptors were killed by scFv(FRP5)-ETA but were resistant to scFv(225)-ETA, indicating that scFv-ETA toxicity is mediated via selective binding to the respective receptor molecules.

11.5 Factors Influencing Toxin Efficacy

The in vitro sensitivity of a target cell for the antibody toxin directed to ErbB-2, and most likely also to other ErbB family members, is influenced by both the amount and the turnover of the receptor. Cells expressing high levels of ErbB-2 are quite sensitive to scFv(FRP5)-ETA while cells with low amounts are more resistant (Wels et al. 1992b). We have also observed an increase in scFv(FRP5)-ETA toxicity in EGF-treated SKBR3 human breast carcinoma cells and EGF-treated HC11 mouse mammary epithelial cells expressing a transfected human erbB-2 cDNA (Wels et al. 1995a). This is likely due to the fact that EGF treatment of cells leads to the formation of activated ErbB-2 and EGF receptor heterodimers which show an increased rate of internalization (Kornilova et al. 1992). Similarly, HC11 mouse mammary epithelial cells transfected with a human erbB-2 cDNA carrying an activating point mutation in the transmembrane domain of the receptor are more sensitive to treatment with scFv(FRP5)-ETA than HC11 cell expressing normal human ErbB-2 protein (Wels et al. 1992b). Activated ErbB-2 has a markedly reduced half-life in HC11 cells when compared to its normal cellular counterpart, suggesting that the rapid internalization of toxin–receptor complexes leads to the increased cytotoxic activity of scFv(FRP5)-ETA on such cells.

The two recombinant toxins specific for the EGF receptor have also proven useful in analyzing factors which influence cellular sensitivity to a toxin. ScFv(225)-ETA displays potent in vitro cell killing activity on cells which overexpress the EGF receptor (Table 1; Wels et al. 1995a). The corresponding growth factor toxin TGF-α-ETA has also been examined for its toxicity on various tumor cell lines. SKBR3 cells express high levels of ErbB-2 and moderate amounts of EGF receptor. The cells are sensitive to low concentrations of the ErbB-2 specific toxin, scFv(FRP5)-ETA, and to TGF-α-ETA, but resistant to high concentrations of scFv(225)-ETA as shown in Fig. 2 and summarized in Table 1.

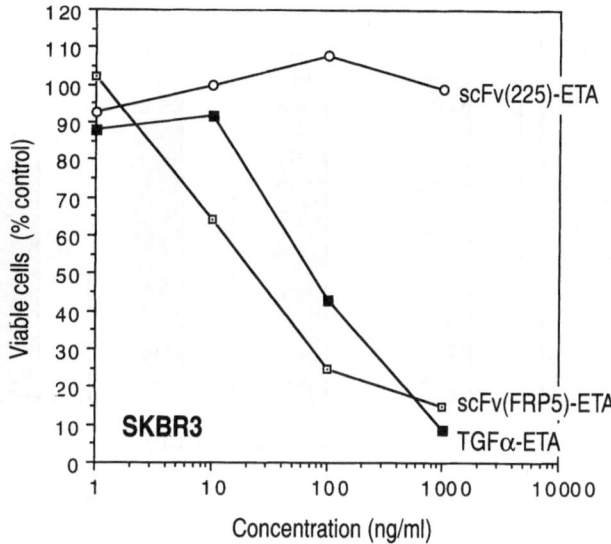

Fig. 2. Inhibition of the in vitro growth of SKBR3 human breast tumor cells by recombinant single-chain toxins. The cells were incubated for 40 h with the indicated concentrations of scFv(225)-ETA (*circles*), transforming growth factor-α *Pseudomonas* exotoxin A (*TGF-α-ETA*) (*closed squares*), or with scFv(FRP5)-ETA (*open squares*). The relative number of viable cells was determined using an enzymatic assay as described (Wels et al. 1992) and is indicated as the absorption at 590 nm. Each *point* was determined in triplicate

These results can be explained by considering the cross-talk between the EGF receptor and ErbB-2. The TGF-α-ETA induces the formation of activated EGF receptor – ErbB-2 heterodimers which are rapidly internalized. ScFv(225)-ETA does not induce EGF receptor activation. In contrast, this antibody toxin competes with activating ligands for binding to the EGF receptor and is therefore restricted to passive internalization via normal EGF receptor turnover (Wels et al. 1995a). This might not allow the intracellular accumulation of an amount of toxin sufficient for cell killing and might restrict its activity to cells expressing very high levels of the target receptor. As expected, A431 human squamous carcinoma cells which overexpress the EGF receptor are sensitive to low concentrations of both EGF receptor-directed toxins. Despite the fact

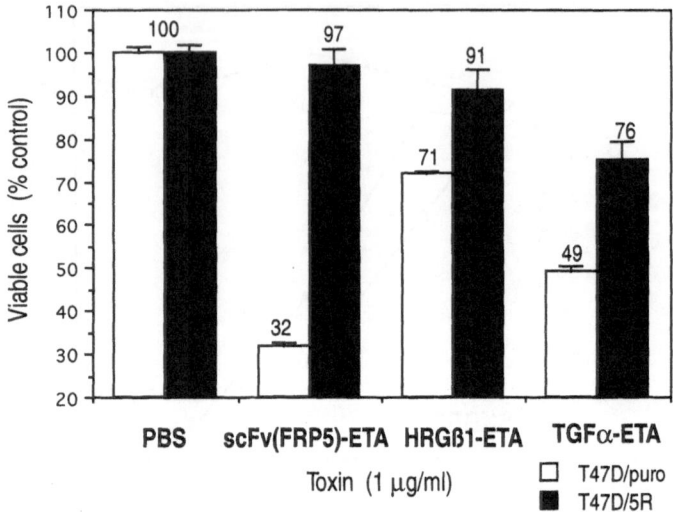

Fig. 3. Sensitivity of T47D/5R human breast tumor cells to recombinant single-chain toxins. T47D/5R cells in which the transit of ErbB-2 to the cell surface is blocked via intracellular expression of the scFv(FRP5) molecule in the endoplasmic reticulum and T47D/puro control cells were treated for 40 h with 1 µg/ml of scFv(FRP5)-ETA, HRGβ1-ETA, or transforming growth factor-α *Pseudomonas* exotoxin A (*TGF-α-ETA*) as indicated. The relative number of viable cells was determined as described in Fig. 2. Each *point* was determined in triplicate. The standard deviation is represented by *error bars*

that the A431 cells have only 10–20,000 ErbB-2 molecules per cell, they are very sensitive to scFv(FRP5)-ETA. A431 cells produce TGF-α, which is released into the culture supernatant and activates EGF receptor in an autocrine fashion (Van de Vijver et al. 1991). It is likely that the TGF-α-induced activation of ErbB-2 through the formation of heterodimers with EGF receptor influences ErbB-2-receptor turnover in these cells and may account for the high sensitivity of A431 cells towards the ErbB-2-specific toxin.

The growth factor toxin HRGβ1-ETA, which contains the receptor-binding domain of the ErbB-3/ErbB-4 ligand heregulin, is highly cytotoxic for tumor cells expressing ErbB-3 and/or ErbB-4 (Jeschke et al. 1995; summarized in Table 1). Following binding of the toxin to HC11 mouse mammary epithelial cells transfected with a human erbB-2 cDNA, there is an increase in the phosphotyrosine content of a protein corresponding in size with ErbB-2; however, HRGβ1-ETA is not cytotoxic for these cells which express only moderate levels of ErbB-3 (Jeschke et al. 1995). Similar to the formation of ligand-induced heterodimers of EGF receptor with ErbB-2 (Goldman et al. 1990; Wada et al. 1990) heterodimerization of ErbB-3 or ErbB-4 with ErbB-2 (Plowman et al. 1993; Sliwkowski et al. 1994), as well as ErbB-3 with EGF receptor (Soltoff et al. 1994), has been reported. The latter might play a role for HRGβ1-ETA activity in A431 cells which are moderately sensitive for this toxin but express only low levels of ErbB receptor tyrosine kinases other than EGF receptor (Table 1).

No natural ligand which binds directly to the ErbB-2 protein is available. However, ErbB-2 is able to form heterodimers with all other ErbB receptor tyrosine kinases upon ligand binding and is activated via receptor transphosphorylation. At least in some cell lines ErbB-2/EGF receptor dimers appear to represent a class of very high affinity receptors for EGF (Wada et al. 1990). Recently it was shown that ErbB-2 can play a critical role in the ligand binding (Karunagaran et al. 1996) and the ligand-induced activation of the other ErbB receptor tyrosine kinases (Graus-Porta et al. 1995; Beerli et al. 1994a). Therefore, depending on the cellular context, ErbB-2 might modulate both the affinity of receptor dimers to natural ligands and the transduction of signals into the cell via different downstream substrates. ErbB-2 receptor heterodimerization is also important for the activity of antibody and growth factor toxins specific for different members of the ErbB receptor tyrosine kinase family. This is exemplified by an experiment using T47D human breast carcinoma cells which naturally express low to moderate levels of the four ErbB receptor proteins. T47D/5R cells were derived by infection of T47D cells with a retroviral construct which directs the intracellular expression of the ErbB-2 specific single-chain antibody scFv(FRP5) to the endoplasmic reticulum (Beerli et al. 1994a; Graus-Porta et al. 1995). This prevents the transit of ErbB-2 to the cell surface but does not affect other ErbB receptor proteins. As expected T47D/5R cells but not control cells infected with the empty retroviral vector became resistant to high concentrations of the antibody-toxin scFv(FRP5)-ETA (Fig. 3). In addition, the sensitvity of T47D/5R cells to HRGβ1-ETA and TGF-α-ETA was also drastically reduced, suggesting that heterodimers of ErbB-2 with ErbB-3 and/or ErbB-4, and of ErbB-2 with EGF receptor play a role in the binding and/or internalization of these toxins.

11.6 Strategies to Improve Toxin Efficacy

ErbB-2 and EGF receptors are often coexpressed in human tumors and have been shown to synergize in the transformation of cells in experimental model systems. In rodent cells coexpression of Neu, the rat ErbB-2 homologue, with EGF receptor leads to the synergistic transformation of cells (Kokai et al. 1989). This is abolished if EGF receptor is coexpressed with kinase-deficient Neu proteins (Qian et al. 1994). The functional interaction of different ErbB receptors might offer the possibility to improve the efficacy of recombinant toxins by administering toxin combinations selected for the individual tumor type. Simultaneous treatment of A431 cells with scFv(FRP5)-ETA and scFv(225)-ETA leads to an additive cytotoxic effect in these cells (Wels et al. 1995a). Another way to target both receptors concurrently is to combine two different binding domains with the toxin moiety in a single polypeptide chain.

We have recently described a novel bivalent, bispecific single chain antibody toxin which contains the scFv(FRP5) and scFv(225) domains fused to truncated ETA (Schmidt et al. 1996). This scFv$_2$(FRP5/225)-ETA protein displays cell-killing activity on tumor cells overexpressing either ErbB-2 or the EGF receptor similar to that of the corresponding monospecific toxins but is more potent in the inhibition of the growth of A431 cells expressing both receptors. In contrast to the monospecific toxins, treatment of A431 cells with scFv$_2$(FRP5/225)-ETA leads to an increase in EGF receptor and ErbB-2 phosphotyrosine content most likely via the induction of receptor heterodimers. This may mechanistically explain the enhanced toxicity of the bispecific antibody toxin. The unique ability of the bispecific molecule to bind simultaneously to both target receptors, thereby inducing the formation of predetermined receptor heterodimers, is also demonstrated by the experiment shown in Fig. 4. The ErbB-2 overexpressing MDA-MB453 breast carcinoma cells were treated for 10 min at 37°C with bispecific scFv$_2$(FRP5/225)-ETA, with monospecific scFv(FRP5)-ETA, or with TGF-α-ETA. Cell lysates were assayed for their phosphotyrosine content by immunoblotting with

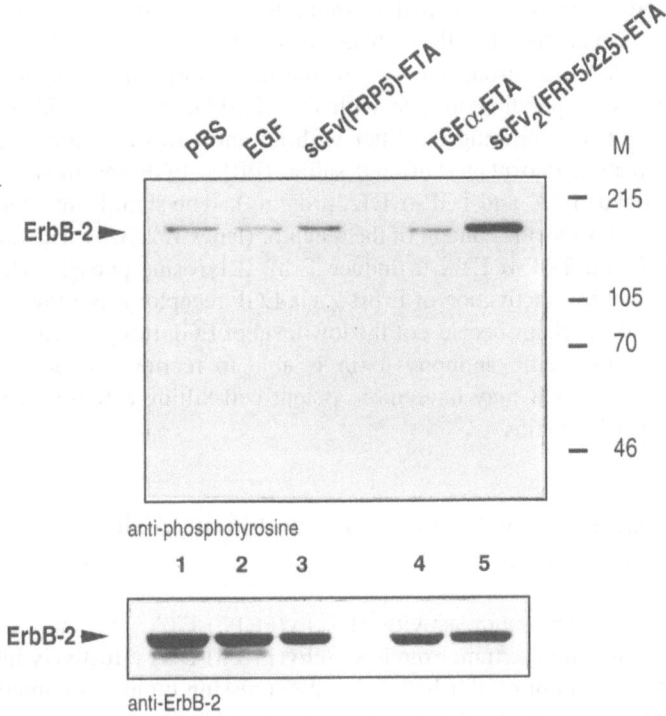

Fig. 4. ScFv2(FRP5/225)-ETA-induced tyrosine phosphorylation of ErbB-2. MDA-MB453 human breast carcinoma cells were grown in low serum for 16 h and then incubated with 1 µg/ml scFv(FRP5)-ETA (*lane 3*), transforming growth factor-α *Pseudomonas* exotoxin A (*TGF-α-ETA; lane 4*), or scFv2(FRP5/225)-ETA (*lane 5*) for 10 min. Control cells were treated with phosphate-buffered saline (*PBS; lane 1*) or 100 ng/ml epidermal growth factor (*EGF; lane 2*). Equal amounts of cell lysates were analyzed by sodium dodecyl sulfate polyacrylamide gel electrophoresis and immunoblotting with an anti-phosphotyrosine monoclonal antibody, followed by incubation with an anti-mouse horseradish peroxidase labeled antibody and chemiluminescent detection (*upper panel*). The amount of ErbB-2 loaded in each *lane* was analyzed by reincubation of the filter with 21N ErbB-2 specific antiserum (*lower panel*). The position of the 185 kDa ErbB-2 protein is indicated. *M*, molecular weight standards

a specific anti-phosphotyrosine antibody. The results are shown in Fig. 4. Treatment of cells with the bispecific scFv$_2$(FRP5/225)-ETA (lane 5) led to a strong increase in the phosphotyrosine content of a protein corresponding in size with the 185-kDa ErbB-2, which was confirmed by reprobing the filter with an anti-ErbB-2 serum (Fig. 4, lower panel). Phosphate-buffered saline (PBS), EGF, the monovalent scFv(FRP5)-ETA, and TGF-α-ETA proteins had no significant effect on the phosphotyrosine content of the receptor (lanes 1, 2, 3, 4). The failure of EGF and TGF-α-ETA to induce ErbB-2 tyrosine phosphorylation shows that transactivation of ErbB-2 via EGF receptor is not favored in these cells, perhaps because of the low level of EGF receptor. Nevertheless, the bispecific antibody toxin is able to recruit both receptors, suggesting that it may have more potent cell-killing activity than the monospecific toxins.

11.7 Antitumoral Activity of Recombinant Toxins in In Vivo Models

The in vivo antitumor activity of scFv(FRP5)-ETA was analyzed in several nude mouse tumor models. ScFv(FRP5)-ETA effectively inhibited the growth of established, ErbB-2-expressing tumors (summarized in Table 2). No unspecific toxicity was observed. The tumors analyzed include: SKOV3 human ovarian carcinoma xenografts (Wels et al. 1992b), A431 human squamous cell carcinoma xenografts (Wels et al. 1995a), and NIH 3T3 mouse fibroblasts transformed by an activated human erbB-2 cDNA (Wels et al. 1995b). Despite a short (30-min) half-life in the circulation of mice, daily treatment with low doses of scFv(FRP5)-ETA, ranging from 1 to 10 µg for a total of 8–10 days, led to a marked reduction in tumor size (Table 2). Systemic treatment with scFv(FRP5)-ETA via intraperitoneal injection as well as continuous infusion from subcutaneously implanted miniosmotic pumps were effective. In adults ErbB-2 is expressed at low levels in epithelial tissues, including gastrointestinal, respiratory, reproductive, urinary tract, skin and breast (Press et al. 1990). The antibody toxin scFv(FRP5)-ETA does not recognize the rodent ErbB-2. Therefore the question of systemic toxicity of this molecule on normal tissues expressing low ErbB-2 levels cannot be addressed in mice or rats.

Table 2. Inhibition of tumor cell growth in vivo by scFv(FRP5)-ETA

*Tumor	ErbB-2 expression[a]	Treatment[b] dose (μg)	Total (% control)[c]	Tumor size
SKOV3[d]	+++++	1 μg/day s.c. days 10–17 p.i.	8μg	36
		6 μg/day s.c. days 10–17 p.i.	48 μg	13
A431 d)	+	10 μg/day i.p. days 6–15 p.i.	100 μg	44
NIH/3T3 #3.7[e] ++		6 μg/day s.c. days 0–7 p.i.	48 μg	20
		6 μg/day s.c. days 4–11 p.i.	48 μg	55*

The antitumoral activity of scFv(FRP5)-ETA in vivo was analyzed in Balb/c athymic nude mice.

[a]Determined by quantitative Western blot experiments.

[b]s.c., Continuous infusion from subcutaneously implanted miniosmotic pumps; p.i., post implantation; i.p., intraperitoneal injection.

[c]Determined 10 days after the end of treatment in comparison to mock-treated animals.

[d]25 mg of established tumor tissue was transplanted on day 0. Treatment was begun when tumor volumes reached approximately 100 mm^3 (Wels et al. 1992b, 1995a).

[e]2×10^6 murine fibroblasts transformed by an activated human erbB-2 allele were injected s.c. on day 0 (Wels et al. 1995b).

The potency of HRGβ1-ETA in inhibiting tumor cell growth in vivo was evaluated in athymic nude mice carrying established ErbB-3 over-expressing MAXF 1162 human mammary carcinoma xenografts (Jeschke et al. 1995). HRGβ1-ETA exhibited strong antitumor activity. A significant, dose-dependent inhibition of MAXF 1162 tumor cell growth was observed in animals treated for 15 days with 0.2 and 0.4 mg/kg/day of HRGβ1-ETA. The strongest antitumor effect was observed during the first week of treatment. During this time transient weight loss and liver toxicity were noted. The toxicity is HRG specific since scFv(FRP5)-ETA which does not recognize mouse receptors did not cause damage to the liver at two times higher concentrations. Moreover, pretreatment of mice with HRG prior to the administration of the fusion protein reduced the weight loss (Jeschke, unpublished observation). ErbB-3 is moderately expressed in several tissues, including brain and liver (Culouscou et al. 1993). Moreover, erbB-4 mRNA has been detected in brain, kidney and heart (Plowman et al. 1993). Our data

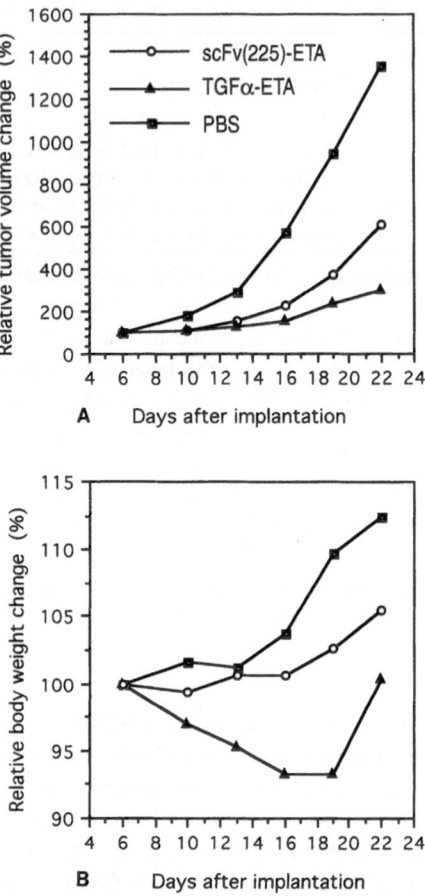

Fig. 5A,B. Effect of recombinant single-chain toxins on the in vivo growth of A431 tumor xenografts in nude mice. A431 tumor tissue (25 mg) was implanted subcutaneously into each mouse (five mice/group). Six days later the mice received i.p. injections of 80 pmol transforming growth factor-α *Pseudomonas* exotoxin A (TGF-α-ETA) (*triangles*) or scFv(225)-ETA (*circles*) twice daily for 10 days. The control group received phosphate-buffered saline (*PBS; squares*). Tumor size (**A**) and body weight (**B**) were measured at the indicated times and tumor volumes were calculated. The mean values for each group are shown

indicate that systemic treatment with heregulin toxins could lead to damage of normal tissues expressing high levels of the target receptors, which could limit the dose of recombinant toxin.

The in vivo antitumor activity of scFv(225)-ETA and TGF-α-ETA was tested on A431 xenografts in nude mice, similar to a previous study focusing on scFv(225)-ETA (Wels et al. 1995a). A431 tumor tissue (25 mg) was implanted s.c. into three groups of five mice on day 0. Six days later when the tumors had reached approximately 100 mm^3 in size treatment was begun. The mice received twice daily intraperitoneal injections of 80 pmol of scFv(225)-ETA (5.3 µg) or TGF-α-ETA (3.8 µg) for a total of 10 days. Control mice received PBS. The results are shown in Fig. 5. Treatment with both fusion toxins led to the inhibition of A431 tumor growth during treatment, with TGF-α-ETA being more effective. By day 22 when the experiment was terminated, the size of the tumors in the scFv(225)-ETA- and TGF-α-ETA-treated animals was 42% and 22% of the tumor size in the control group, respectively. A transient weight loss was observed during the course of the TGF-α-ETA treatment (Fig. 5b). The animals recovered quickly after the end of the treatment, indicating that at the dose chosen systemic toxicity is not severe.

Some normal tissues including hepatocytes express significant numbers of EGF receptor which could complicate the administration of TGF-α-containing toxins in vivo (Real et al. 1986). Systemic treatment of mice with high doses of TGF-α-PE40, a fusion toxin very similar to the TGF-α-ETA used in this study, resulted in fatal liver damage, thus limiting the amount of toxin which could be applied safely (Pai et al. 1991). In a recent clinical study of TGF-α-PE40 (TP40) in superficial bladder cancer, the molecule was administered directly into the bladder by transurethral instillation in order to avoid systemic toxicity (Goldberg et al. 1995). The treatment was well tolerated by the patients, indicating that local treatment, where applicable, might circumvent systemic toxicity. Alternatively the use of an antibody-derived cell recognition domain instead of a growth factor domain might allow the safe administration of recombinant EGF receptor-specific toxins in humans. As shown above, at least in vitro scFv(225)-ETA activity is restricted to cells which highly overexpress EGF receptor, whereas TGF-α-ETA is also cytotoxic for cells expressing only moderate levels of the receptor.

11.8 Conclusions

Members of the ErbB family of receptor tyrosine kinases are potent signal-transducing molecules whose activation stimulates numerous intracellular pathways which are likely to be important in tumor cell growth. The extracellular accessibility of these receptors provides a target for cytotoxic molecules. The differential expression of the receptors, high on the surface of tumor cells and low in normal epithelial tissues, makes it possible to design toxic molecules which preferentially recognize tumor cells and provides a rational for the further development of such reagents for clinical applications. Novel insights into the biology of the ErbB receptor tyrosine kinases and their functional interaction can be translated into improved therapeutic approaches. However, the practical application of these molecules in the clinic is still preceeded by extensive preclinical toxicity studies. Systemic therapy with ErbB-targeted antibody or growth factor toxins could have unforeseen side effects in humans.

The progress in such diverse areas of research such as molecular oncology, tumor immunology, molecular biology, and biotechnology converges in the development of new therapeutic modalities. In the near future it will become possible to "individualize" cancer therapy, i.e., to exploit the biochemical characteristics of the cancer cells of individual patients and administer drugs which act specifically on these cells. This might diminish the current side effects of cytotoxic drugs and increase the success rate of the treatment.

Acknowledgments. We wish to thank Dr. J. Mendelsohn for making the 225 hybridoma cell line available to us. This work was supported in part by a grant from the Deutsche Forschungsgemeinschaft (SFB 364-C1) and a fellowship by the Schweizerischer Nationalfonds zur Förderung der wissenschaftlichen Forschung for M. Hoffmann.

References

Beerli RR, Wels W, Hynes NE (1994a) Intracellular expression of single chain antibodies reverts ErbB-2 transformation. J Biol Chem 269:23931–23936

Beerli RR, Wels W, Hynes NE (1994b) Autocrine inhibition of the epidermal growth factor receptor by intracellular expression of a single-chain antibody. Biochem Biophys Res Commun 204:666–672

Culouscou JM, Plowman GD, Carlton GW, Green JM Shoyab M (1993) Characterization of a breast cancer cell differentiation factor that specifically activates the HER4/p180erbB4 receptor. J Biol Chem 268:18407–18410

Ennis BW, Valverius EM, Bates SE, Lippman ME, Bellot F, Kris R, Schlessinger J, Masui H, Goldenberg A, Mendelsohn J, Dickson RB (1989) Anti-epidermal growth factor receptor antibodies inhibit the autocrine-stimulated growth of MDA-468 human breast cancer cells. Mol Endocrinol 3:1830–1838

Fan Z, Mendelsohn J, Masui H, Kumar R (1993) Regulation of epidermal growth factor receptor in NIH3T3/HER14 cells by antireceptor monoclonal antibodies. J Biol Chem 268:21073–21079

Goldberg MR, Heimbrook DC, Russo P, Sarosdy MF, Greenberg RE, Giantonio BJ, Linehan WM, Walther M, Fisher HAG, Messing E, Crawford ED, Oliff AE, Pastan IH (1995) Phase I clinical study of the recombinant oncotoxin TP40 in superficial bladder cancer. Clin Cancer Res 1:57–61

Goldman R, Ben Levi R, Peles E, Yarden Y (1990) Heterodimerization of the erbB-1 and erbB-2 receptors in human breast carcinoma cells: a mechanism for receptor transregulation. Biochemistry 29:11024–11028

Graus-Porta D, Beerli RR, Hynes NE (1995) Single-chain antibody-mediated intracellular retention of ErbB-2 impairs neu differentiation factor and epidermal growth factor signaling. Mol Cell Biol 15:1182–1191

Gullick WJ (1991) Prevalence of aberrant expression of the epidermal growth factor receptor in human cancers. Br Med Bull 47:87–98

Harwerth, IM, Wels W, Marte BM, Hynes NE (1992) Monoclonal antibodies against the extracellular domain of the erbB-2 receptor function as partial ligand agonists. J Biol Chem 267:15160–15167

Harwerth IM, Wels W, Schlegel J, Müller M, Hynes NE (1993) Monoclonal antibodies directed to the erbB-2 receptor inhibit in vivo tumour cell growth. Br J Cancer 68:1140–1145

Hudziak RM, Lewis GD, Winget M, Fendly BM, Shepard HM, Ullrich A (1989) p185HER2 monoclonal antibody has antiproliferative effects in vitro and sensitizes human breast tumor cells to tumor necrosis factor. Mol Cell Biol 9:1165–1172

Hynes NE, Stern DF (1994) The biology of erbB-2/neu/HER-2 and its role in cancer. Biochem Biophys Acta 1198:165–184

Jeschke M, Wels W, Dengler W, Imber R, Stöcklin E, Groner B (1995) Targeted inhibition of tumor cell growth by recombinant heregulin-toxin fusion proteins. Int J Cancer 60:730–739

Karunagaran D, Tzahar E, Beerli RR, Chen X, Graus-Porta D, Wen D, Seger R, Hynes NE, Yarden Y (1996) ErbB-2 is a common auxiliary subunit of NDF- and EGF-receptors: implications for breast cancer. EMBO J 15:254–264

Kasprzyk PG, Song SU, DiFiore PP, King CR (1992) Therapy of an animal model of human gastric cancer using a combination of anti-erbB-2 monoclonal antibodies. Cancer Res 52:2771–2776

Kawamoto T, Sato JD, Le A, Polikoff J, Sato GH, Mendelsohn J (1983) Growth stimulation of A431 cells by epidermal growth factor: identification of high-affinity receptors for epidermal growth factor by an anti-receptor monoclonal antibody. Proc Natl Acad Sci USA 80:1337–1341

Kokai Y, Myers JN, Wada T, Brown VI, LeVea CM, Davis JG, Dobashi K, Greene MI (1989) Synergistic interaction of p185c-neu and the EGF receptor leads to transformation of rodent fibroblasts. Cell 58:287–292

Kornilova ES, Taverna D, Hoeck W, Hynes NE (1992) Surface expression of erbB-2 protein is post-transcriptionally regulated in mammary epithelial cells by epidermal growth factor and by the culture density. Oncogene 7:511–519

Lemoine NR, Barnes DM, Hollywood DP, Hughes CM, Smith P, Dublin E, Prigent SA, Gullick WJ, Hurst HC (1992) Expression of the ERBB3 gene product in breast cancer Br J Cancer 66:1116–1121

Masui H, Kawamoto T, Sato JD, Wolf B, Sato G, Mendelsohn J (1984) Growth inhibition of human tumor cells in athymic nude mice by anti-epidermal growth factor receptor monoclonal antibodies. Cancer Res 44:1002–1007

Moritz D, Wels W, Mattern J, Groner B (1994) Cytotoxic T lymphocytes with a grafted recognition specificity for erbB-2 expressing tumor cells. Proc Natl Acad Sci USA 91:4318–4322

Pai LH, Gallo MG, FitzGerald DJ, Pastan I (1991) Antitumor activity os a transforming growth factor α-Pseudomonas exotoxin fusion protein (TGF-α-PE40). Cancer Res 51:2808–2812

Pastan I, FitzGerald D (1991) Recombinant toxins for cancer treatment. Science 254:1173–1177

Peles E, Yarden Y (1993) Neu and its ligands: from an oncogene to neural factors. Bioessays 15:815–824

Plowman GD, Green JM, Culouscou JM, Carlton GW, Rothwell VM, Buckley S (1993) Heregulin induces tyrosine phosphorylation of HER4/p180erbB4. Nature 366:473–475

Press MF, Cordon-Cardo C, Slamon DJ (1990) Expression of the HER-2/neu proto-oncogene in normal human adult and fetal tissues. Oncogene 5:953–962

Qian X, Dougall WC, Hellman ME, Greene MI (1994) Kinase-deficient neu proteins suppress epidermal growth factor receptor function and abolish cell transformation. Oncogene 9:1507–1514

Real F, Rettig W, Chesa P, Melamed MR, Old LJ, Mendelsohn J (1986) Expression of epidermal growth factor receptor in human cultured cells and tissues: relationship to cell lineage and stage of differentiation. Cancer Res 46:4726–4731

Schmidt M, Hynes NE, Groner B, Wels W (1996) A bivalent single-chain antibody-toxin specific for ErbB-2 and the EGF receptor. Int J Cancer 65:538–546

Siegall CB, Xu YH, Chaudhary VK, Adhya S, FitzGerald D, Pastan I (1989) Cytotoxic activities of a fusion protein comprised of TGFα and Pseudomonas exotoxin. FASEB J 3:2647–2652

Sliwkowski MX, Schaefer G, Akita RW, Lofgren JA, Fitzpatrick VD, Nuijens A, Fendly BM, Cerione RA, Vandlen RL, Carraway KL III (1994) Coexpression of erbB2 and erbB3 proteins reconstitutes a high affinity receptor for heregulin. J Biol Chem 269:14661–14665

Soltoff SP, Carraway KL III, Prigent SA, Gullick WG, Cantley LC (1994) ErbB3 is involved in activation of phosphatidylinositol 3-kinase by epidermal growth factor. Mol Cell Biol 14:3550–3558

Stancovski I, Hurwitz E, Leitner O, Ullrich A, Yarden Y, Sela M (1991) Mechanistic aspects of the opposing effects of monoclonal antibodies to the ERBB2 receptor on tumor growth. Proc Natl Acad Sci USA 88:8691–8695

Tzahar E, Levkowitz G, Karunagaran D, Yi L, Peles E, Lavi S, Chang D, Liu N, Yayon A, Wen D, Yarden Y (1994) ErbB-3 and ErbB-4 function as the respective low and high affinity receptors of all neu differentiation factor/heregulin isoforms J Biol Chem 269: 25226–25233

Van De Vijver MJ, Kumar R, Mendelsohn J (1991) Ligand-induced activation of A431 cell epidermal growth factor receptors occurs primarily by an autocrine pathway that acts upon receptors on the surface rather than intracellularly. J Biol Chem 266:7503–7508

Wada T, Qian X, Greene MI (1990) Intermolecular association of the p185neu protein and the EGF receptor modulates EGF receptor function. Cell 61:1339–1347

Wels W, Harwerth IM, Hynes NE, Groner B (1992a) Diminution of antibodies directed against tumor cell surface epitopes: a single chain Fv fusion molecule specifically recognizes the extracellular domain of the c-erbB-2 receptor. J Steroid Biochem Mol Biol 43:1–7

Wels W, Harwerth IM, Müller M, Groner B, Hynes NE (1992b) Selective inhi-
    bition of tumor cell growth by a recombinant single-chain antibody-toxin
    specific for the erbB-2 receptor. Cancer Res 52:6310–6317
Wels W, Harwerth IM, Zwickl M, Hardman N, Groner B, Hynes NE (1992c)
    Construction, bacterial expression and characterization of a bifunctional
    single-chain antibody-phosphatase fusion protein targeted to the human
    erbB-2 receptor. Biotechnology 10:1128–1132
Wels W, Beerli R, Hellmann P, Schmidt M, Marte BM, Kornilova ES, Hekele
    A, Mendelsohn J, Groner B, Hynes NE (1995a) EGF receptor and
    p185erbB-2 specific single-chain antibody-toxins differ in their cell killing
    activity on tumor cells expressing both receptor proteins. Int J Cancer
    60:137–144
Wels W, Moritz D, Schmidt M, Jeschke M, Hynes NE, Groner B (1995b)
    Biotechnological and gene therapeutic strategies in cancer treatment. Gene
    159:73–80
Winter G, Milstein C (1991) Man-made antibodies. Nature 349:293–299
Zdanovsky AD, Chiron M, Pastan I, FitzGerald DJ (1993) Mechanism of ac-
    tion of Pseudomonas exotoxin. Identification of a rate-limiting step. J Biol
    Chem 268:21791–21799

12 EGF Receptor Inhibition by Antibody as Anticancer Therapy

J. Mendelsohn, J. Baselga, X. Wu, D. Peng, C. Brown,
J.L. Chou, H. Masui, and Z. Fan

12.1 Background

Many human epithelial tumors (approximately one of three) have been found to express high numbers of epidermal growth factor (EGF) receptors, and increased receptor levels are associated with a poor clinical prognosis in cancers involving the bladder (Neal et al. 1985; Harris et al. 1989), breast (Sainsbury et al. 1985; Harris et al. 1989), and lung (Veale et al. 1987; Hendler et al. 1989). Furthermore, EGF receptor activation has been implicated in autocrine stimulation of cell growth in many experimental studies (Mendelsohn 1990). Therefore, the EGF receptor appears to be an excellent target for antitumor therapy (Mendelsohn 1989).

12.2 Inhibition of EGF Receptor Tyrosine Kinase by a Monoclonal Antibody Inhibits Cell Proliferation in Culture and in Xenografts

We have produced and characterized two monoclonal antibodies (mAbs) against the human EGF receptor, 225 IgG1, and 528 IgG2a (Kawamoto et al. 1983; Sato et al. 1983). They bind to the receptor with affinity similar to the natural ligands, EGF and transforming growth factor-α (TGF-α), compete with ligands for receptor binding, and inhibit ligand-induced activation of receptor tyrosine kinase (Kawamoto et al. 1983, 1984; Sato et al. 1983; Gill et al. 1984). These effects of antireceptor mAb are demonstrated in Fig. 1 (Fan et al. 1993c). Both bivalent 225 mAb and the 225 Fab' monovalent fragment can inhibit binding of labeled EGF to membranes from A431 squamous carcinoma cells, and binding depends on the molar ratio of EGF and mAb. Figure 1B shows the capacity of bivalent and high quantities of monovalent 225 mAb to inhibit the activation of HER14 cell EGF receptors by exogenous TGF-α. HER14 is an NH-3T3 cell line transfected with the human EGF receptor, which was selected for study because it produces no endogenous TGF-α (kindly provided by J. Schlessinger). The mAbs have been shown to inhibit proliferation of a variety of cultured epithelial tumor cell lines that express EGF receptors and TGF-α, including skin (vulva) (Kawamoto et al. 1983, 1984; Sato et al. 1983; Mendelsohn 1990), breast (Arteaga et al. 1988; Ennis et al. 1989), colon (Masui et al. 1991; Karnes et al. 1992; Wu et al. 1995), lung (Reiss et al. 1992), kidney (Atlas et al. 1992), and prostate (Hofer et al. 1991) cells. Even more pronounced growth inhibition was observed when the mAbs were added to cultures of nontransformed cells (Sato et al. 1983; Markowitz et al. 1990; Chou et al. 1996). Inhibition of cell growth has been suggested to result from blockade of EGF receptor activation by growth factor either present in the culture medium or produced by the cells in an autocrine fashion, since treatment with anti-EGF receptor mAbs that did not block binding of ligand was unable to inhibit growth (Sato et al.

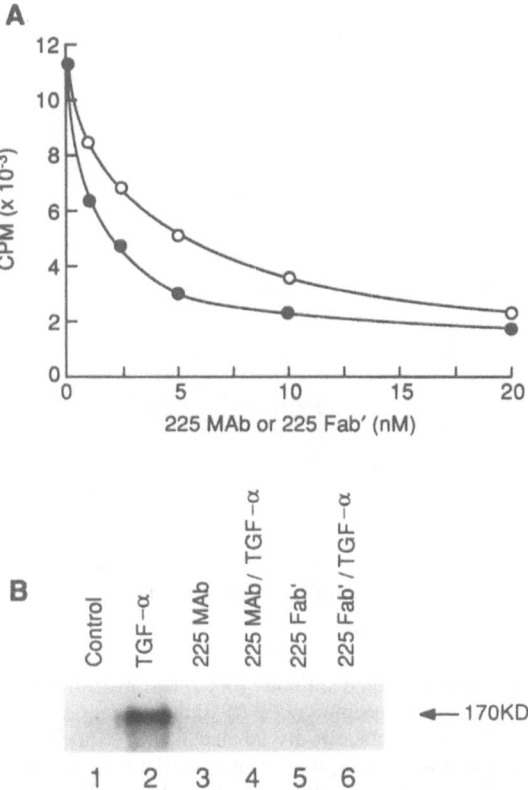

Fig. 1A,B. Characteristics of bivalent 225 monoclonal antibody (*mAb*) and monovalent 225 *Fab'*. **A** Epidermal growth factor (*EGF*) receptor binding competition assay. A431 cell membranes were plated as described in Sect. 12.2. ^{125}I-labeled EGF (5 n*M*) plus indicated concentrations of 225 mAb (*closed circles*) or 225 Fab' (*open circles*) were added to the wells. Cell membranes were incubated on ice for 2 h, and the associated radioactivity was measured in a -counter. Each *point* represents the average of duplicate determinations after subtracting the background, obtained by adding 100-fold excess unlabeled EGF. **B** Assay of tyrosine phosphorylation. HER14 cells were cultured with additions of 10 n*M* transforming growth factor- (*TGF-*), 200 n*M* 225 mAb, and 1000 n*M* 225 Fab' as indicated for 30 min at 37°C and lysed with sodium dodecyl sulfate (SDS) sample buffer. The lysates were boiled and resolved by 7% SDS polyacrylamide gel electrophoresis and immunoblotted with anti-phosphotyrosine antibody PY69

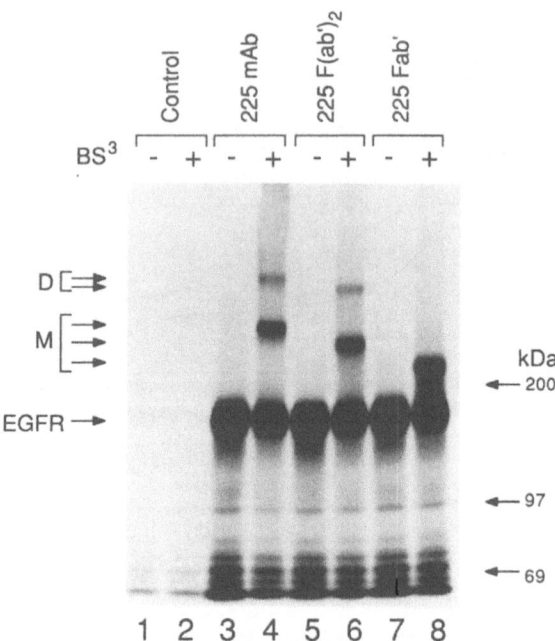

Fig. 2. Capacity of monoclonal antibody (*mAb*) and mAb fragments to induce epidermal growth factor receptor (*EGFR*) dimerization. A431 cells (5×105 cells/20-mm dish) were metabolically labeled with [^{35}S]methionine for 16 h. The cells were prechilled on ice for 15 min and the labeling medium was replaced with medium containing 100 nM 225 mAb, 225 F(ab')2, or 225 Fab', followed by incubation for 1 h on ice. Cells were then washed twice with cold phosphate-buffered saline and incubated on ice with or without 3 mM BS3 cross-linker (bis[sulfosuccinimidyl]suberate; *BS*) for 20 min with gentle shaking. The cross-linking was quenched by the addition of 10 mM ammonium acetate (final concentration) and cells were lysed with RIPA buffer. Lysates containing equal amounts of protein were subjected to immunoprecipitation in the presence of rabbit anti-mouse antibody. The precipitates were resolved by 3%–7% gradient nonreducing sodium dodecyl sulfate polyacrylamide gel electrophoresis followed by autoradiography. *D*, dimer; *M*, monomer

1983; Mendelsohn et al. 1987; Markowitz et al. 1990; Van de Vijver et al. 1991).

While both monovalent 225 Fab' and bivalent 225 mAb can block EGF receptor activation by exogenous ligand, we found that the bivalent form is far more successful in blocking both receptor kinase activation and A431 cell proliferation stimulated by endogenous TGF-α (Fan et al. 1994). It also was found that bivalent mAb is far more effective than monovalent mAb in downregulating EGF receptors. These effects were attributed to the capacity of bivalent 225 mAb, but not monovalent 225 Fab', to produce receptor dimerization (without activating kinase activity; Fig. 2; Fan et al. 1994).

Why should the bivalent 225 mAb be more successful than monovalent 225 Fab' in inhibiting A431 cell proliferation? The answer to this question may lie in our observations on the prevalence of membrane-bound TGF-α in these cells. Soluble TGF-α is derived from pro-TGF-α, a 20- to 22-kDa transmembrane precursor (Derynck et al. 1984; Lee et al. 1985) which undergoes several post-translational modifications that include N-and O-linked glycosylation. In transfected fibroblasts, maturation of pro-TGF-α in the plasma membrane involves two sequential enzymatic digestions. First, the rapid cleavage of an N-terminal portion by pro-TGF—ase-I leaves a cell-associated 17-kDA pro-TGF-α form that still contains the mature sequence of TGF-α (Derynck et al. 1984; Teixido and Massague 1988). The second cleavage by pro-TGF–ase II is slower and results in release of the 6-kDa soluble TGF-α fragment, leaving behind a cell-associated 15-kDa residual terminal fragment, often referred to as a tail.

In pulse-labeling studies with Chinese hamster ovary (CHO) cells transfected with human TGF-α we observed that this process of sequential enzymatic cleavage goes to near completion in 4 h. Most of the TGF-α precursor found in these cells after 4 h is the 15-kDa tail (Fig. 3; Baselga et al. 1996). However, in the case of A431 cells and a number of other malignant cell lines, TGF-α accumulates predominantly in the 17-kDa transmembrane form, while the amount of 15-kDa tail is modest, even after 4 h of culture. This suggests that in the malignant cell lines tested, the membrane-anchored pro-TGF-α form represents a significant portion of biosynthesized TGF-α. It is possible that this membrane-bound form of the ligand could carry out juxtacrine stimulation of EGF receptors on adjacent cells, or even receptors on adjacent portions

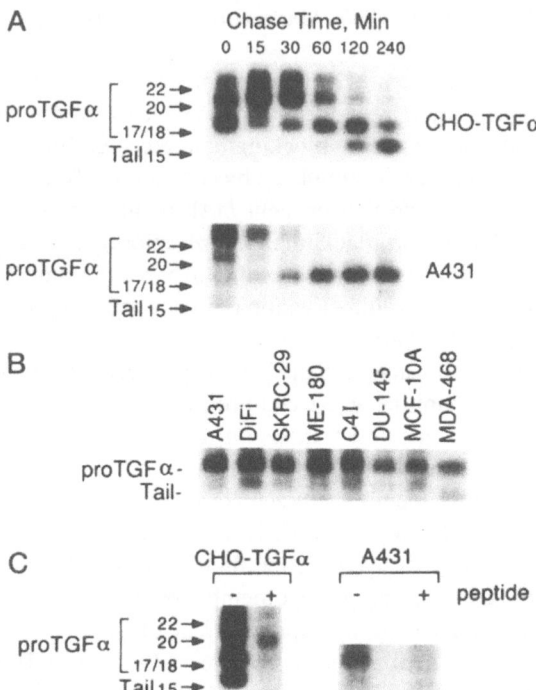

Fig. 3A–C. Molecular forms of transforming growth factor- (*TGF-*) in tumor cell lines expressing EGF receptors. **A** Chinese hamster ovary (*CHO-TGF-*) and A431 cells were metabolically labeled with [^{35}S]cysteine for 30 min and chased for the depicted time periods. Pro-TGF- was immunoprecipitated from cell lysates with rabbit anti-pro-TGF- antibodies (directed at a pro-TGF-COOH-terminal sequence). Immunocomplexes were processed by sodium dodecyl sulfate polyacrylamide gel electrophoresis and analyzed by autoradiography. The molecular weights of the different growth factor species are shown at the *left*. **B** A panel of malignant cell lines known to express the EGF receptor was analyzed for pro-TGF- expression 4 h after metabolic labeling as above. Cell lines include: A431 squamous carcinomas; DiFi colon carcinoma; SKRC-29 renal cell carcinoma; ME-140 and C4I cervix carcinoma; DU-145 prostate carcinoma; MCF-10A nonmalignant breast cells; MDA-468 breast carcinoma. **C** Immunoprecipitations were performed in the presence of an excess (1 m*M*) of competing peptide against which the anti-pro-TGF- antibody was raised. The competing peptide prevented immunoprecipitation of pro-TGF- by the antibody

of the plasma membrane of the same cell. Since the endogenous, membrane-bound TGF-α is present in close proximity to EGF receptors, it may have a competitive advantage over an antireceptor mAb in the culture medium. However, if the mAb, in bivalent form, were able to downregulate the receptor, this would effectively remove the receptor from access to ligand. This could explain why bivalent mAb, which cross-links and subsequently downregulates EGF receptor, is more effective in inhibiting cell growth than monovalent Fab', which does not cause receptors to dimerize and downregulate.

In vivo effects of treatment with anti-EGF receptor mAbs were assayed using xenografts of human tumors in athymic mice. Administration of receptor-saturating concentrations of either 225 IgG1 or 528 IgG2a mAb intraperitoneally for 3 weeks, beginning within a few days of tumor cell implantation subcutaneously, caused a dose-dependent, durable inhibition of tumor growth (Masui et al. 1984). Successful prevention of tumor growth was achieved against breast and bowel adenocarcinoma cell lines, cervical and vulvar squamous tumor cell lines, and renal cell cancer (Masui et al. 1984, 1991; Mendelsohn et al. 1987; Atlas et al. 1992; Fan et al. 1993a). An F(ab')$_2$ 225 fragment administered in vivo could produce nearly comparable antitumor activity (Fan et al. 1993a). Experiments with ^{111}In-labeled mAb demonstrated that anti-EGF receptor mAb could selectively image tumor xenografts bearing elevated levels of EGF receptors (Goldenberg et al. 1989). We postulate that the characteristic defining tumor cell susceptibility to antibody is production of TGF-α and response to it in an autocrine fashion (Mendelsohn et al. 1987). It should be noted that the evidence for physiologic effects of anti-EGF receptor mAbs upon receptor activation does not rule out possible concurrent activity of these antibodies as immune effector agents in vivo.

While therapy with 225 mAb can successfully prevent the growth of human tumor xenografts in nude mice treated within a week of inoculation, treatment fails to eliminate well-established xenografts of most tumor cell lines tested (Masui et al. 1984). An exception is the DiFi colorectal adenocarcinoma cell line, which displays the highest sensitivity to mAb 225 of all cell lines that we have studied. Well-established xenografts of DiFi cells are completely eradicated after mAb treatment (Masui et al. 1991).

12.3 Biochemical Mechanism of Anti-EGF Receptor mAb-Mediated Inhibition of Cell Proliferation Involves Inhibition of Cyclin-Dependent Kinase Activity

Progression through different cell cycle stages is regulated at a series of checkpoints, at which both external and internal signals are integrated into the cell cycle (Hunter and Pines 1994). The checkpoint regulating progression of cells through G1 phase and into S phase is controlled by a family of cyclin-dependent kinases (CDKs) and their corresponding activating partners, the cyclins (Hunter and Pines 1994). In mammalian cells, the main cyclin–CDK complexes are cyclin D-CDK4/CDK6, cyclin E-CDK2, and cyclin A-CDK2, acting primarily in middle to late G1 phase, the G1/S phase boundary, and S phase, respectively. Progression through G1 phase requires orderly activation of these different CDKs (Sherr 1994). One of the critical substrates of G1 CDKs is the retinoblastoma protein (Rb), whose phosphorylation and subsequent release of Rb-bound transcription factors such as E2F are required for G1 to S phase transition (Sherr 1994).

We began our studies of the mechanism of antireceptor mAb in experiments with DiFi cells, because of their exquisite sensitivity to EGF receptor blockade. When these cells are exposed to saturating concentrations of 225 mAb, the cultures accumulate in G1 phase (Wu et al. 1995, 1996). Under these conditions Rb remains hypophosphory-lated (Wu et al. 1995). To explore the mechanism of this inhibition we assayed the amount and activity of the CDK associated with Rb phosphorylation during traversal from G1 to S phase of the cell cycle. CDK activity was assayed with histone H1 substrate in immunoprecipitates from DiFi cells formed with anti-cyclin E, anti-cyclin A, or anti-CDK2 antibody. We observed that addition of 225 mAb to cultures produced marked kinase inhibition within 24 h. In contrast, there was little change in the activity of CDK6 or CDK4 kinases, measured using GST-Rb as substrate (Wu et al. 1996).

To determine the explanation for the reduced CDK2 kinase activity we first measured the amounts of CDK2, cyclin E, and cyclin A by western blotting and found no decrease in protein levels in cells treated with 225 mAb (Wu et al. 1996). We then assayed inhibitors of CDK and found that 225 mAb stimulated a two- to threefold increase in the level of p27KIP1 protein. The increased p27KIP1 was found to be associated with CDK2, but not CDK4/6. Furthermore, removal of p27KIP1 from cell extracts could deplete them of inhibitory activity against CDK2. Changes in the amount of p21WAF1 were not observed.

The observation that 225 mAb-induced accumulation of cells in G1 phase was accompanied by elevated levels of p27KIP1 inhibitor of CDK activity in DiFi colon adenocarcinoma cells was followed by similar findings in studies with A431 squamous carcinoma cells (Fan et al. 1996), DU145 prostate adenocarcinoma cells, (Peng et al. 1996), and the immortalized but nonmalignant breast cell line MCF10A (Chou et al. 1996). In the malignant cell lines, except for DiFi, G1 arrest was never complete in response to 225 mAb-mediated EGF receptor blockade, whereas 98% of mAb-treated malignant MCF10A cells accumulated in G1 phase. In these cell lines, cyclin D levels and CDK6 activity were also found to be modified to varying degrees, which had not been the case for DiFi cells. Thus p27KIP1-mediated inhibition of CDK activity appears to be a generalized response to blockade of EGF-receptor kinase by antireceptor antibody. It was noted that DiFi cells are uniquely sensitive to deprivation from EGF receptor kinase activity. In fact, receptor blockade in cultures of these cells eventually results in activation of programmed cell death. These epithelial cells appear to be unique auxotrophs for TGF-α/EGF. All other cells studied either arrested completely in G1 phase (nonmalignant cells) or slowed growth with accumulation in G1 phase (malignant cells) in response to EGF receptor blockade, but did respond to receptor blockade with loss of viability.

12.4 Combination Therapy with Anti-EGF Receptor mAb Plus Chemotherapy Results in Enhanced Cytotoxicity Against Tumor Cell Xenografts

For therapy, we wished to augment the efficacy of anti-EGF receptor mAb so that antitumor activity could be obtained against well-established xenografts. We noted a report that treatment with cisplatinum enhanced the activity of a single dose of another anti-EGF receptor mAb in preventing growth of a tumor xenograft (Aboud-Pirak et al. 1988). This stimulated us to systematically test the effect of combining 225

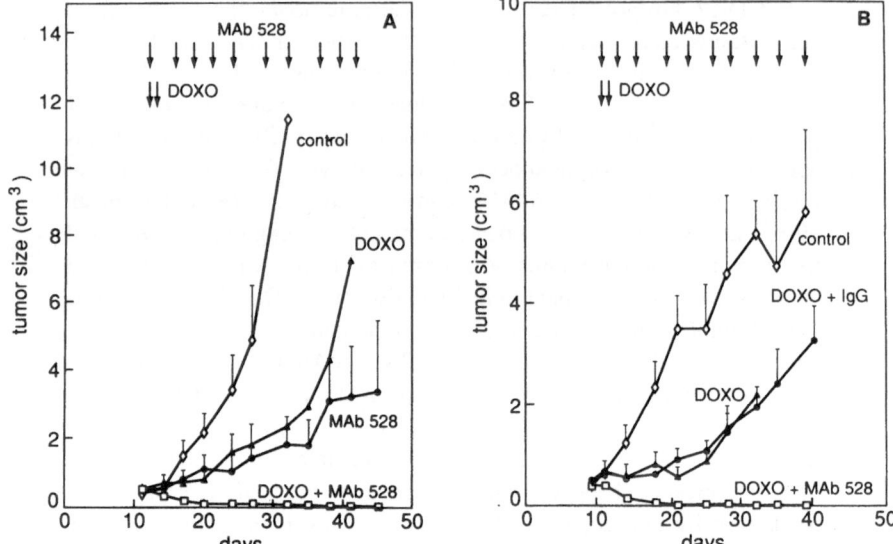

Fig. 4A,B. Antitumor activity of monoclonal antibody 528 (*MAb 528*) in combination with doxorubicin (*DOXO*) on well-established A431 squamous cell carcinoma xenografts in athymic mice. Treatment was started when tumors reached a mean size of 0.4 cm³ on day 11. Each treatment group consisted of at least five animals. Results are given in mean tumor size ± SE. *Error bars* are not present when less than three animals remained alive in a certain treatment group. Doxorubixin (100 µg/20 g body weight) was given intraperitoneally on days 1 and 2 of treatment (day 11 and 12 or day 9 and 10 after tumor cell inoculation). mAb 528 (1 mg) was given intraperitoneally on day 1 of treatment and twice a week thereafter for a total of ten doses. **A** Treatment with either doxorubicin alone or mAb alone partially inhibited tumor growth. Doxorubicin in combination with mAb 528 completely eradicated all tumors in the animals surviving on day 30 (*n*=8). B) Doxorubicin in combination with a nonspecific mouse IgG did not result in a greater antitumor effect than doxorubicin alone. While doxorubicin in combination with mAb 528 resulted in disappearance of all tumors in the animals surviving on day 30 (*n*=6). *Arrows* show days on which treatment was administered

mAb treatment with the chemotherapeutic agents most commonly used against epithelial malignancies.

Experiments with A431 cell cultures and xenografts explored the anti-tumor effects of combined therapy with doxorubicin and anti-EGF receptor mAb (Baselga et al. 1993). Culture of A431 squamous carcinoma or MDA-468 adenocarcinoma cells with doxorubicin at various concentrations (0–10 nM), in combination with 528 mAb or 225 mAb, produced additive inhibition of growth in both tumor cell lines, increasing the inhibitory effects of doxorubicin by up to 42%. The increased anti-tumor activity was not observed when cultured cells were treated with doxorubicin in combination with the nonblocking anti-EGF receptor 455 mAb. We then explored the effects of the combination therapy against tumor xenografts of these two cell lines. When tumors reached approximately 0.4 cm^3, mice were allocated into groups with comparable tumor sizes and intraperitoneal therapy was started. In untreated animals, tumors grew rapidly and all of the animals had to be sacrified within 5 weeks, as expected (Fig. 4; Baselga et al. 1993). Doxorubicin alone in the maximum tolerated dose slowed tumor growth, but within 10 days tumors began to regrow rapidly. Treatment with optimal doses of 528 mAb (1 mg twice a week) reduced tumor growth; however, as expected from previous studies with well-established tumors, the xenografts were not eliminated. In contrast, the combination treatment with doxorubicin and 528 mAb resulted in a major anti-tumor effect, with tumor elimination in all of the animals. Experiments with 225 mAb in combination with doxorubicin gave similar results. Treatment with a control nonspecific IgG given in combination with doxorubicin resulted in no change in tumor growth, compared with doxorubicin alone.

Parallel studies were carried out using 225 mAb or 528 mAb in combination with the maximum tolerated dose of cisplatinum. In these studies against well established A431 cell xenografts, mAb alone or cisplatinum alone had insubstantial effects, but combination therapy again produced cures in tumor-bearing mice that were followed for over 6 months (Fig. 5; Fan et al. 1993b).

A third series of experiments was carried out with paclitaxel against MDA468 breast adenocarcinoma cells. In this case, the tumors were quite sensitive to paclitaxel therapy, and suboptimal drug doses were used to assess the effect of concurrent 225 mAb. The results again

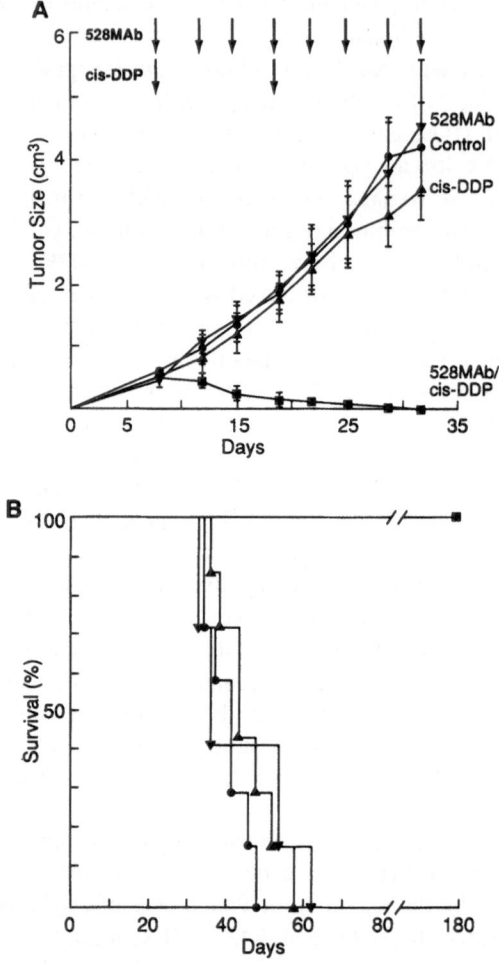

Fig. 5A,B. Eradication of A431 cell xenografts by combination treatment with
monoclonal antibody 528 (*MAb 528*) and cis-diamminedichloroplatinum (*cis-DDP*). A431 cell (10^7) were implanted s.c. into nude mice and allowed to grow
for 8 days. In **A**, the mice were given i.p. injections of either phosphate-buff-
ered saline (*circles*); two injections of cis-DDP (150 µg/25 g mouse weight) on
day 8 and day 18 (*triangles up*); or mAb 528, 1 mg/mouse, twice a week for
4 weeks, with (*squares*) or without (*triangles down*) two injections of cis-DDP
(150 µg/25 g mouse weight) on day 8 and day 18. *Arrows*, the timing of drug
and antibody treatment. The data are expressed as the mean tumor size ± SE
(seven mice per group). In **B**, the mice were observed for 6 months for survival

demonstrated elimination of well established xenografts by combined treatment (J. Baselga et al., unpublished observation).

These experiments with adenocarcinoma and squamous carcinoma xenografts demonstrated the efficacy of combining EGF receptor blockade (528 or 225 mAb) with cytotoxic chemotherapy (doxorubicin, cisplatinum, or paclitaxel). The mechanisms of these additive effects are under investigation in our laboratory. In studies with collaborators, we have preliminary evidence that addition of 225 mAb may prolong the period of recovery from biochemical injury produced by cisplatin or doxorubicin, and this type of interaction may indeed explain our observations. However, we favor an alternative interpretation of our findings, which implicates checkpoint regulation of the cell cycle as the activator of cell death in this model.

Traversal through the cell cycle is biochemically maintained at checkpoints, two of which in late G1 phase and prior to M phase appear to be the most significant. When cells are functioning properly, deprivation from the signaling pathway activated by essential growth factors activates the G1 checkpoint and cells arrest in G1 phase. Likewise, cells damaged by chemotherapy arrest typically in G2/M or G1 phase, in order to repair alterations in DNA, tubulin, or other molecules. Malignant cells appear to be able to disobey checkpoints without jeopardizing cell survival, as is seen with most tumor cells exposed to 225 mAb in culture. However, we hypothesize that when tumor cells simultaneously disobey two checkpoint signals (activated by 225 mAb plus chemotherapy), this is intolerable and results in cell death. Another way of conceptualizing this is to consider that in the face of chemotherapeutic damage, which signals the cell to pause for repair, the requirement for a growth factor in order to proliferate (traverse the cell cycle) is converted to requirement of the growth factor for survival. Thus, malignant epithelial cells damaged by chemotherapy now act like DiFi cells, and when deprived of EGF receptor kinase activity they can no longer survive. There is ample precedent for growth factors acting as survival factors in hematopoietic cell lines, in cultures of nerve cells, and in epithelial cells driven to proliferate by constitutive expression of myc (reviewed in Meikrantz and Schlegel 1995).

In summary, we hypothesize that combined treatment with anti-EGF receptor mAb plus chemotherapy may have enhanced antitumor activity due to the simultaneous activation of dual checkpoints, which are disobeyed by the tumor cells. A correlary of this hypothesis is the prediction that nonmalignant epithelial cells, which obey the checkpoint signals, will be less susceptible to cytotoxicity from this combination therapy. Furthermore, hematopoietic cells do not express EGF receptors. Thus, we postulate a novel method for intensifying the effect of chemotherapy without requiring rescue by bone marrow stem cells. In our model, selective dose intensification against malignant epithelial cells is achieved by addition of EGF receptor blockade.

12.5 Clinical Trials with Anti-EGF Receptor mAb 225

Our hypothesis is being tested in clinical trials with patients with advanced cancer. In the initial clinical study, murine 225 mAb was administered successively in escalating single intravenous doses to patients with advanced squamous carcinoma of the lung, a tumor that invariably expresses high levels of EGF receptors (Divgi et al. 1991). The antibody was labeled with ^{111}In, to permit pharmacological and nuclear scanning studies. The results showed:

1. Marked uptake of mAb 225 in the liver (presumably Kupffer cells and hepatocytes)
2. Visualization by gamma camera of primary tumors and all metastases larger than 1 cm in diameter (by CT scan or X-ray) with 225 mAb doses of 40 mg or more
3. Achievement of serum levels of mAb adequate to saturate EGF receptors (20 nM) with doses of 100 mg or more
4. Safety at doses of mAb 225 up to 300 mg, without changes in blood tests measuring liver and kidney function
5. Human anti-mouse antibodies (HAMA) detected at 2 weeks

This was followed by a phase I studies with a human chimeric form of the antibody, designated C225. These studies utilized unlabeled antibody. Escalating doses were administered to different subjects, first as single intravenous infusions and then, in a current study, as repeated weekly infusions for up to 12 doses. Saturating levels could be maintained by weekly doses of 100 mg/m^2 without evidence of toxicity. There was stabilization of disease in a number of the patients receiving repeated doses of antibody (Bos et al. 1996). No anti-human immune responses were detected in the single dose study, and the multiple dose trial has yet to be analyzed.

Phase IB/IIA clinical trials have been initiated to test combination therapy with C225 plus chemotherapy in patients with tumors expressing high levels of EGF receptors. Eligible patients will be treated with:

1. C225 plus doxorubicin for advanced prostatic cancer
2. C225 plus cisplatinum for advanced head and neck and lung cancer
3. C225 plus paclitaxel for breast cancer

12.6 Summary

We have demonstrated the capacity of a mAb to block activation of signal transduction from EGF receptors. Combination therapy with anti-EGF receptor mAb plus chemotherapy is effective against well established human tumor xenografts. This novel form of combination therapy may be useful in a large number of patients with epithelial malignancies.

We hypothesize that the mechanism of action of combined therapy with C225 mAb and chemotherapy involves simultaneous activation of two checkpoints regulating cell cycle progression, resulting in activation of cell death in the malignant cells.

References

Aboud-Pirak E, Hurwitz E, Pirak ME, Bellot F, Schlessinger J, Sela M (1988) Efficacy of antibodies to epidermal growth factor receptor against KB carcinoma in vitro and in nude mice. J Natl Cancer Inst 80:1605–1611

Arteaga CL, Coronado E, Osborne CK (1988) Blockade of the epidermal growth factor receptor inhibits transforming growth factor-alpha-induced but not estrogen-induced growth of hormone-dependent human breast cancer. Mol Endocr 2:1064–1069

Atlas I, Mendelsohn J, Baselga J, Masui H, Fair WR, Kumar R (1992) Growth regulation of human renal carcinoma cells: role of transforming growth factor-alpha. Cancer Res 52:3335–3339

Baselga J, Norton L, Masui H, Pandiella A, Coplan K, Cordon-Cardo C, Miller W, Mendelsohn J (1993) Anti-tumor effects of doxorubicin in combination

with anti-epidermal growth factor receptor monoclonal antibodies. J Natl
Cancer Inst 85:1327–1331

Baselga J, Mendelsohn J, Kim Y-M, Pandiella A (1996) Autocrine regulation
of membrane transforming growth factor-alpha cleavage. J Biol Chem
271:3279–3284

Bos M, Mendelsohn J, Bowden C, Pfister D, Cooper MR, Cohen R, Burtness
B, D'Andrea G, Waksal H, Norton L, Baselga J (1996) Phase I studies of
anti-epidermal growth factor receptor chimeric monoclonal antibody C225
in patients with EGFR overexpressing tumors. Am Soc Clin Oncol 15:443
(abstract no 1381)

Chou JL, Fan Z, Koff A, Mendelsohn J (1996) EGF receptor blockage induces
reversible growth arrest and changes in proteins that regulate the cell cycle
in human mammary epithelial cells. Proc Am Assoc Cancer Res 37:10 (abstract no 68)

Derynck R, Roberts AB, Winkler ME, Chen EY, Goeddel DV (1984) Human
transforming growth factor-: precursor structure and expression in E. coli.
Cell 38:287–297

Derynck R, Goeddel DV, Ullrich A, Gutterman JU, Williams RD, Bringman
TS, Berger WH (1987) Synthesis of messenger RNAs for transforming
growth factors alpha and beta and the epidermal growth factor receptor by
human tumors. Cancer Res 47:707–712

Divgi CR, Welt C, Kris M, Real FX, Yeh SDJ, Gralla R, Merchant B,
Schweighart S, Unger M, Larson SM, Mendelsohn J (1991) Phase I and imaging trial of indium-111 labeled anti-EGF receptor monoclonal antibody
225 in patients with squamous cell lung carcinoma. J Natl Cancer Inst
83:97–104

Ennis BW, Valverius EM, Lippman ME, Bellot F, Kris R, Schlessinger J,
Masui H, Goldenberg A, Mendelsohn J, Dickson RB (1989) Monoclonal
anti-EGF receptor antibodies inhibit the growth of malignant and non-ma-
lignant human mammary epithelial cells. Mol Endocrinol 3:1830–1838

Fan Z, Masui H, Atlas I, Mendelsohn J (1993a) Blockade of epidermal growth
factor (EGF) receptor function by bivalent and monovalent fragments of
225 anti-EGF receptor monoclonal antibody. Cancer Res 53:4322–4328

Fan Z, Baselga J, Masui H, Mendelsohn J (1993b) Antitumor effect of anti-
EGF receptor monoclonal antibodies plus cis-Diaminedichloroplatinum
(cis-DDP) on well established A431 cell xenografts. Cancer Res
53:4637–4642

Fan Z, Mendelsohn J, Masui H, Kumar R (1993c) Regulation of epidermal
growth factor receptor in NIH3T3/HER14 cells by antireceptor monoclonal
antibodies. J Biol Chem 268:21073–21079

Fan Z, Lu Y, Wu X, Mendelsohn J (1994) Antibody-induced epidermal growth factor receptor dimerization mediates inhibition of autocrine proliferation of A431 squamous carcinoma cells. J Biol Chem 269:27595–27602

Fan Z, Shang BY, Wu X, Peng D, Lu Y, Chou J, Koff A, Mendelsohn J (1996) Blockade of epidermal growth factor receptor by anti-EGFR monoclonal antibody 225 causes G1 arrest of A431 cells with induction of p27KIP1. Proc Am Assoc Cancer Res 37:10 (abstract no 69)

Gill GN, Kawamoto T, Cochet C, Le A, Sato JD, Masui H, MacLeod CL, Mendelsohn J (1984) Monoclonal anti-epidermal growth factor receptor antibodies which are inhibitors of epidermal growth factor binding and antagonists of epidermal growth factor-stimulated tyrosine protein kinase activity. J Biol Chem 259:7755–7760

Goldenberg A, Masui H, Divgi C, Kamrath H, Pentlow K, Mendelsohn J (1989) EGF receptor overexpression and localization of nude mouse xenografts using Indium-111 labelled anti-EGF receptor monoclonal antibody. J Natl Cancer Inst 81:1616–1625

Harris AL, Nicholson S, Sainsbury JRC, Neal D, Smith K, Farndon JR, Wright C (1989) Epidermal growth factor receptor: a marker of early relapse in breast cancer and tumor stage progression in bladder cancer; interactions with neu. In: Furth M, Greaves M (eds)The molecular diagnostics of human cancer. Cold Spring Harbor Laboratory Press, Cold Spring Harbor, New York, pp 353–357

Hendler F, Shum-Siu A, Nanu L, Yuan D, Ozanne B (1989) Increased EGF receptors and the absence of an alveolar differentiation marker predict a poor survival in lung cancer. Proc Am Clin Oncol 8:223 (abstract no 869)

Hofer DR, Sherwood ER, Bromberg WD, Mendelsohn J, Lee C, Kozlowski JM (1991) Autonomous growth of androgen-independent human prostatic carcinoma cells: role of transforming growth factor-α. Cancer Res 51:2780–2785

Hunter T, Pines J (1994) Cyclins and cancer. II: cyclin D and CDK inhibitors come of age. Cell 79:573–582

Karnes WEJ, Walsh JH, Wu SV, Kim RS, Martin MG, Wong HC, Mendelsohn J, Gazdar AF, Cuttitta F (1992) Autocrine stimulation of EGF receptors by TGF-αalpha regulates autonomous proliferation of human colon cancer cells. Gastroenterology 102:474–485

Kawamoto T, Sato JD, Le A, Polikoff J, Sato GH, Mendelsohn J (1983) Growth stimulation of A431 cells by EGF: identification of high affinity receptors for epidermal growth factor by an anti-receptor monoclonal antibody. Proc Natl Acad Sci USA 80:1337–1341

Kawamoto T, Mendelsohn J, Le A, Sato GH, Lazar CS, Gill GN (1984) Relation of epidermal growth factor receptor concentration to growth of human epidermoid carcinoma A431 cells. J Biol Chem 259:7761–7766

Lee DC, Rose TM, Webb NR, Todaro GJ (1985) Cloning and sequence analysis of a cDNA for rat transforming growth factor-α. Nature 313:489–491

Markowitz SD, Molkentin K, Gerbic C, Jackson J, Stellato T, Willson JKV (1990) Growth stimulation by coexpression of transforming growth factor-alpha and epidermal growth factor receptor in normal and adenomatous human colon epithelium. J Clin Invest 86:356–362

Masui H, Kawamoto T, Sato JD, Wolf B, Sato GH, Mendelsohn J (1984) Growth inhibition of human tumor cells in athymic mice by anti-EGF receptor monoclonal antibodies. Cancer Res 44:1002–1007

Masui H, Boman B, Hyman J, Castro L, Mendelsohn J (1991) Treatment with anti-EGF receptor monoclonal antibody causes regression of DiFi human colorectal carcinoma xenografts. Proc Am Assoc Cancer Res 32:394 (abstract no 2340)

Meikrantz W, Schlegel R (1995) Apoptosis and the cell cycle. J Cell Biochem 58:160–174

Mendelsohn J (1989) Potential clinical applications of anti-EGF receptor monoclonal antibodies. In: Furth, M, Greaves M (eds) Cancer cells. Cold Spring Harbor Laboratory Press, Cold Spring Harbor, New York, pp 359–362

Mendelsohn J (1990) The epidermal growth factor receptor as a target for therapy with antireceptor monoclonal antibodies. Semin Cancer Biol 1:339–344

Mendelsohn J, Masui H, Goldenberg A (1987) Anti-epidermal growth factor receptor monoclonal antibodies may inhibit A431 tumor cell proliferation by blocking on autocrine pathway. Trans Assoc Am Phys 100:173–178

Neal DE, Bennett MK, Hall RR, Marsh C, Abel PD, Sainsbury JRC, Harris AL (1985) Epidermal growth factor receptors in human bladder cancer: comparison of invasive and superficial tumors. Lancet 1:366–368

Peng D, Fan Z, Lu Y, DeBlasio T, Scher H, Mendelsohn J (1996) Blockade of epidermal growth factor receptor by anti-EGFR monoclonal antibody (mAb225) induces G1 arrest in prostatic cancer cell line DU145. Proc Am Assoc Cancer Res 37:243 (abstract no 1664)

Reiss M, Stash EB, Vellucci VF, Zhou Z-I (1992) Activation of the autocrine transforming growth factor alpha pathway in human squamous carcinoma cells. Cancer Res 51:6254–6262

Sainsbury JRC, Malcolm AJ, Appleton DR, Farndon JR, Harris AL (1985) Presence of epidermal growth factor receptor as an indicator of poor prognosis in patients with breast cancer. J Clin Pathol 38:1225–1228

Sato JD, Kawamoto T, Le AD, Mendelsohn J, Polikoff J, Sato GH (1983) Biological effect in vitro of monoclonal antibodies to human EGF receptors. Mol Biol Med 1:511–529

Sherr CJ (1994) G1 phase progression: cycling on cue. Cell 79:551–555

Teixido J, Massague J (1988) Structural properties of a soluble bioactive precursor for transforming growth factor-α. J Biol Chem 263:3924–3929

Van de Vijver M, Kumar R, Mendelsohn J (1991) Ligand-induced activation of A431 cell EGF receptors occurs primarily by an autocrine pathway that acts upon receptors on the surface rather than intracellularly. J Biol Chem 266:7503–7508

Veale D, Ashcroft T, Marsh C, Gibson GJ, Harris AL (1987) Epidermal growth factor receptors in non-small cell lung cancer. Br J Cancer 55:513–516

Wu X, Fan Z, Masui H, Rosen N, Mendelsohn J (1995) Apoptosis induced by an anti-epidermal growth factor receptor monoclonal antibody in a human colorectal carcinoma cell line is inhibited by insulin. J Clin Invest 95:1897–1905

Wu X, Rubin M, Fan Z, DeBlasio T, Soos T, Koff A, Mendelsohn J (1996) Involvement of p27KIP1 in G1 arrest mediated by an anti-epidermal growth factor receptor monoclonal antibody. Oncogene 12:1397–1403

Subject Index

Ernst Schering Research Foundation Workshop

Editors: Günter Stock
Ursula-F. Habenicht

This series will be available on request from
Ernst Schering Research Foundation, 13342 Berlin, Germany